CLINICAL WARD

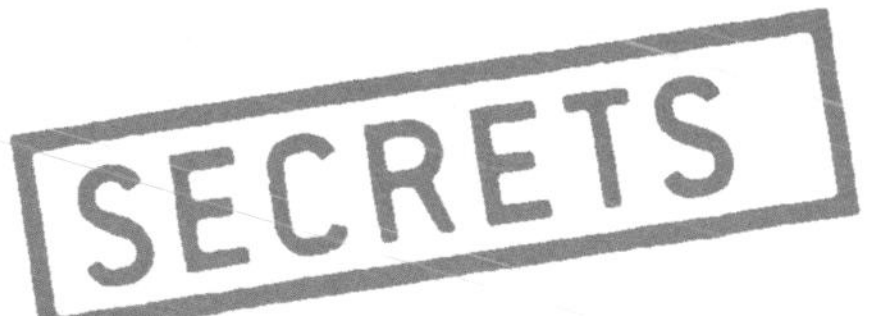

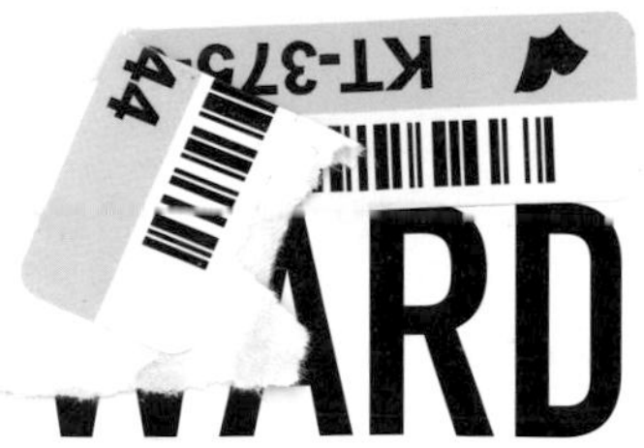

CLINICAL WARD

SECRETS

Mitesh S. Patel
MD/MBA, Class of 2009
University of Michigan Medical School
The Wharton School, University of Pennsylvania

Derek K. Juang
MD, Class of 2008
University of Michigan Medical School

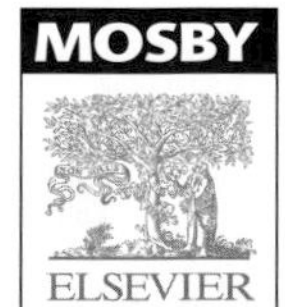

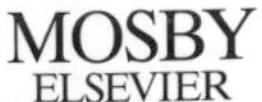

1600 John F. Kennedy Blvd.
Ste 1800
Philadelphia, PA 19103-2899

CLINICAL WARD SECRETS ISBN: 978-0-323-05750-9

Notice

Knowledge and best practice in this field are constantly changing. As new research and experience broaden our knowledge, changes in practice, treatment and drug therapy may become necessary or appropriate. Readers are advised to check the most current information provided (i) on procedures featured or (ii) by the manufacturer of each product to be administered, to verify the recommended dose or formula, the method and duration of administration, and contraindications. It is the responsibility of the practitioner, relying on their own experience and knowledge of the patient, to make diagnoses, to determine dosages and the best treatment for each individual patient, and to take all appropriate safety precautions. To the fullest extent of the law, neither the Publisher nor the Authors assume any liability for any injury and/or damage to persons or property arising out of or related to any use of the material contained in this book.

The Publisher

Library of Congress Cataloging-in-Publication Data

Patel, Mitesh S.
Clinical ward secrets / Mitesh S. Patel, Derek K. Juang. — 1st ed.
p. ; cm. — (Secrets series)
Includes bibliographical references and index.
ISBN 978-0-323-05750-9 (alk. paper)
1. Clinical medicine—Handbooks, manuals, etc. 2. Hospital wards—Handbooks, manuals, etc. I. Juang, Derek K. II. Title. III. Series.
[DNLM: 1. Clinical Medicine—education. 2. Hospital Departments—organization & administration. 3. Internship and Residency. 4. Patient Care Management—organization & administration.
WB 18 P295c 2010]
RC55.P365 2010
616—dc22 2008041731

Acquisitions Editor: James Merritt
Developmental Editor: Nicole DiCicco
Project Manager: Mary B. Stermel
Marketing Manager: Allan McKeown

Printed in China

Last digit is the print number: 9 8 7 6 5 4 3 2 1

CONTENTS

CONTRIBUTORS

Nitin K. Gupta
MD, Class of 2008
University of Michigan Medical School

Derek K. Juang
MD, Class of 2008
University of Michigan Medical School

Stephen Y. Kang
MD, Class of 2009
University of Michigan Medical School

Joseph D. Maratt
MD, Class of 2008
University of Michigan Medical School

Mitesh S. Patel
MD/MBA, Class of 2009
University of Michigan Medical School
The Wharton School, University of Pennsylvania

Aditi Saxena
MD, Class of 2008
University of Michigan Medical School

Eric W. Schneider
MD, Class of 2008
University of Michigan Medical School

Javier A. Valle
MD, Class of 2008
University of Michigan Medical School

ACKNOWLEDGMENTS

We would like to thank the following attending physicians for their chapter reviews, suggestions, and help in producing this book.

Michael J. Englesbe, MD
Assistant Professor, Transplant Surgery
University of Michigan Medical School

Laura R. Hopson, MD
Assistant Professor, Emergency Medicine
University of Michigan Medical School

Christopher S. Kim, MD, MBA
Assistant Professor, Internal Medicine
Assistant Professor, Pediatrics and Communicable Diseases
University of Michigan Medical School

Monica L. Lypson, MD
Assistant Dean, Graduate Medical Education
Assistant Professor, Internal Medicine
University of Michigan Medical School

We would like to thank the following colleagues for their chapter reviews, suggestions, and help in producing this book.

Gopi J. Astik
MD, Class of 2008
University of Missouri-Kansas City School of Medicine

Seetharam C. Chadalavada
MD/MS, Class of 2009
Cleveland Clinic Lerner College of Medicine at Case Western Reserve University

George R. Cheely, Jr
MD/MBA, Class of 2009
University of Pennsylvania School of Medicine
The Wharton School, University of Pennsylvania

Andrew T. Evans, JD
MBA, Class of 2009
The Wharton School, University of Pennsylvania

Jason R. Guercio
MD/MBA, Class of 2009
University of Pennsylvania School of Medicine
The Wharton School, University of Pennsylvania

Rebecca D. Kolsky
MD/MBA, Class of 2009
University of Pennsylvania School of Medicine
The Wharton School, University of Pennsylvania

Deepa Kumaraiah
MD/MBA, Class of 2009
University of Pennsylvania School of Medicine
The Wharton School, University of Pennsylvania

Ankit A. Mahadevia
MD/MBA, Class of 2008
The Johns Hopkins School of Medicine
The Wharton School, University of Pennsylvania

Chethra K. Muthiah
MD, Class of 2007
Wright State University Boonshoft School of Medicine

Christopher F. Pirok
MD, Class of 2010
Rush Medical College

Jill A. Schondebare
MD, Class of 2011
University of Connecticut School of Medicine
MBA, Class of 2009
The Wharton School, University of Pennsylvania

Ankur M. Shah
MD, Class of 2006
Northwestern University Feinberg School of Medicine

Ashish R. Shah
MD, Class of 2008
University of Pittsburgh School of Medicine

Niraj S. Shah
MD, Class of 2010
University of Toledo School of Medicine

Rishi K. Sharma
MD, Class of 2008
Wayne State University School of Medicine

We would like to thank the following editors at Elsevier for their hard work and help in producing this book.

James Merritt
Acquisition Editor

Nicole DiCicco
Developmental Editor

To our parents:
Subhash and Hemlata Patel
Jer-nan and Lily Juang

For their love and support
during our journey in medicine

PREFACE

How do I admit a patient to the cardiology service? How do I consult the endocrine department about a patient's diabetic issues? What steps are involved when a patient arrives at the hospital and needs emergent surgery? These are common questions that medical students ask themselves while on the clinical wards. Unfortunately, the answers are often hard to come by. Many common processes within the hospital become second nature to physicians and staff, and therefore are not regularly taught to students. Furthermore, few resources exist for students to find answers to these questions on their own.

Our goal is to help medical students better prepare for the clinical wards. Students often begin their rotations without much preparation or direction. As medical students, we went through a similar situation. Without any helpful resources, we turned to fourth-year medical students for advice. While they provided valuable insights, there was no standard method for collecting their information. Now, as fourth-year medical students having completed more than a year of clinical rotations, we have used our recent experiences to describe the topics we feel are most important for preparation on the clinical wards. This book provides a simple and concise description of hospital operations and is meant to be used as a guide and resource for students on the clinical wards.

Hospitals vary tremendously from institution to institution. Despite this great diversity, many of the everyday basic processes are conducted similarly. To account for as much variation as possible, students from over ten different medical schools have reviewed these chapters to inform us of any differences among institutions. We know it is not possible to create a version of this book that is specifically tailored to every medical school, but we hope that this rigorous review process has made our book applicable to students across the country.

Several staff attending physicians have reviewed chapters in this book. We feel this process has helped to ensure that our discussion of topics is accurate. However, we understand that the medical field is constantly changing. Therefore any content within this book must be taken into perspective with regard to each medical student's unique situation.

This book was written to be composed of two integrated parts. The first part is a discussion of the process of medicine. It begins with an overview of the U.S. healthcare system and then follows a patient through the healthcare system, from arrival in the emergency department to hospital discharge and outpatient follow-up. We suggest that students read this book from front to back to take advantage of this conceptual outline.

The second part of the book includes material that students can reference while on the wards. This material is presented throughout the book. We have also included a chapter on procedures in which students may have the opportunity to participate while on the wards. By referencing these materials prior to rotations, patient encounters, or procedures, we believe that students can be better prepared to learn from their experiences.

We hope medical students will find this book as a valuable resource. We wish it had existed when we began on the clinical wards.

Mitesh S. Patel
Derek K. Juang

TOP 100 SECRETS

These secrets are the top 100 key points to keep in mind while on the clinical boards. They summarize concepts and principles of the U.S. healthcare system and patient care.

1. The major players in the U.S. healthcare system are the providers (e.g., physicians and nurses), payers/insurers (e.g., Medicare and health maintenance organizations [HMO]), and suppliers (e.g., pharmaceutical and medical device companies).

2. The organizational management of a typical hospital is divided into two entities. The hospital administration is organized by a chief executive officer (CEO) and an executive committee to govern the hospital's finance, building and grounds, and public relations committees. The clinical medical staff governs each of the clinical departments such as pediatrics, radiology, and urology.

3. Medicare is a federally funded program that provides insurance to elderly persons age 65 and older, patients with end-stage kidney failure, and some qualified disabled persons.

4. Medicaid is a state and federally funded insurance program that mainly covers patients below certain thresholds of the poverty line. Each individual state's legislature runs the program for its state.

5. The Emergency Medical Treatment and Active Labor Act (EMTALA) of 1986 requires that any patient arriving to the emergency department requesting medical care must be provided an appropriate medical screening examination and subsequent necessary care regardless of ability to pay or lack of insurance.

6. When in the emergency department setting, be sure to check the patient's vital signs to ensure that he or she is stable before taking a history. If the patient appears unstable, find a physician immediately to determine whether emergency action is necessary.

7. When presenting a patient in the emergency department, keep in mind that time is limited and interruptions are frequent. Keep the presentation short and focused. When presenting the differential diagnosis, some find it helpful to think of two parallel (sometimes overlapping) differential diagnoses. Use one differential diagnosis that considers life-threatening possibilities and one that considers the most likely diagnoses.

8. In the emergency department, the "ABCs" stand for Airway, Breathing, and Circulation. It is important to always check these three items first when initially assessing a patient.

9. Contraindications to placing a Foley catheter include blood at the urethral meatus, a scrotal hematoma, a displaced pelvic fracture, and a high riding prostate on rectal examination.

10. FAST stands for focused assessment with sonography in trauma. It is a portable ultrasound machine used to check for intraperitoneal bleeding in trauma patients.

11. In general, nonabsorbable, monofilament sutures (e.g., Ethilon or Prolene) are most suitable for surface wound closure because they cause the least scarring and lowest infection risk. Deep or buried sutures must be absorbable (e.g., Vicryl).

12. When assessing suture sizes for use, 2-0 (pronounced "two-oh") is the thickest and is used for high-tension surfaces such as the knee. A 5-0 or 6-0 suture is generally used for areas with less surface tension such as the face.

13. An emergency discharge summary should be written in a patient-friendly language and reviewed with the patient. It should include a discharge diagnosis, discharge medications, and follow-up instructions.

14. When a patient arrives to the hospital in distress, needs emergency resuscitation or surgery, and is unable to give consent because of the presenting medical condition, the patient may be admitted and treated without consent.

15. The decision of which department a patient is admitted to is most commonly made in the emergency department. The patient's primary symptoms and hospital protocols typically determine which department he or she will go to. However, sometimes the decision is made on the basis of the amount of patients already on each service.

16. The key portions of history-taking include the chief complaint, history of present illness, past medical/surgical history, medications and allergies, family history, social history, review of systems/symptoms, and code status (if the patient is admitted).

17. The key portions of the physical examination include the vital signs, general observation, HEENT (head, eyes, ears, neck, and throat), cardiovascular, pulmonary, abdominal, skin and extremities, genitourinary and rectal, and neurologic.

18. A useful mnemonic for writing admission orders is ADC VAN DIMSL, which stands for Admit to, Diagnosis, Condition, Vital signs, Activity, Nursing, Diet, IV fluids, Meds/allergies, Special circumstances, and Labs.

19. To "staff" a patient means to present the patient's history, physical examination, laboratory results, studies, assessment, and plan to the attending physician who is responsible for the patient's care.

20. An assessment of a new patient should be limited to a few lines of dialogue and should give a summary of the patient's age, sex, significant past medical history, significant risk factors, presenting signs and symptoms, and differential diagnosis. The assessment is also sometimes referred to as the impression.

21. There are two standard methods of organizing the management plan during a patient presentation: a systems-based approach and a problem-based approach. Although the method chosen is usually based on the attending's preference, a problem-based approach is most often used for patients with a few medical issues and a systems-based approach is used for more patients with more complex medical problems such as those in the intensive care unit.

22. The majority of laboratory requests (e.g., simple blood tests) written on inpatient care floors are routine and take 4 to 6 hours on average for processing. Orders can be written as STAT requests, which are processed much faster (e.g., simple blood test results are returned within 1 hour).

23. The most commonly used metabolic panels are the basic and the comprehensive. Each can be used to identify common electrolyte, glucose, and renal abnormalities but the comprehensive panel also includes information on transaminases, total bilirubin levels, and total protein and albumin levels. Synonyms for the basic panel include Chem-8 and SMA-8. Some institutions use the Chem-7, SMA/SMAC-7, and Metabolic Panel 7.

24. A complete blood count assesses red blood cell count, hemoglobin level, hematocrit, red blood cell indices, and white blood cell count. A platelet count can also be requested if necessary.

25. A patient presenting with chest pain typically needs laboratory tests including a basic metabolic panel, complete blood count, and cardiac enzyme measurements, as well as diagnostic tests such as an electrocardiogram and chest x-ray.

26. The gold standard test is the single diagnostic test that is considered to be definitive for a certain disease process and should ideally be close to 100% sensitive and 100% specific. Although the gold standard may be the best test, often it is not the most commonly performed because of invasiveness or high cost.

27. An arterial blood gas (ABG) analysis is most commonly ordered to determine the severity of oxygenation deficit, evaluate hypo- or hyperventilation, evaluate acid-base status, or check the maintenance of patients receiving chronic mechanical ventilation.

28. The ABCDEFGH approach to interpreting chest x-rays stands for Assessment/Airway, Bones/Soft tissue, Cardiac, Diaphragm, Effusions, Fields, Great Vessels, and hila/mediastinum.

29. The "Are There Many Lung Lesions" mnemonic for interpreting chest x-rays stands for Abdomen, Thorax, Mediastinum, Lungs alone, Lungs together.

30. In general, the upper limit for width of the cardiac silhouette on chest x-ray is 50% of the thoracic diameter on an anteroposterior film.

31. An acute abdominal series is a set of x-rays of the upright chest, upright abdomen, and supine abdomen.

32. The medical record is intended to provide a detailed account of the care that a patient receives and is essential for quality and continuity of care. It is also important for billing and legal purposes.

33. The medical record should include the history, physical examination, medical decision-making, the basis for those decisions, and any procedures, laboratory tests, or diagnostic tests.

34. The SOAP format is typically used for a daily progress note. This stands for Subjective, Objective, Assessment, and Plan.

35. An order is a single specific instruction to be implemented according to a patient's medical care protocol and can be executed only once or scheduled to occur at regular intervals.

36. An order can be stopped by writing a discontinuation (D/C) instruction such as "D/C penicillin."

37. When one is writing an order for a medication, it is essential that the following four components are noted in the same sequence each time: [medication name] [dose] [route] [timing/schedule]. It is also possible to specify the number of times that the medication should be administered.

38. The common routes of medication administration include mouth (PO), intravenous (IV), subcutaneous (SC/SubQ), intramuscular (IM), rectal (PR), topical, inhalation, and through a feeding tube.

39. PRN stands for *pro re nata* meaning "as needed" in Latin. An advantage of a PRN order is having a standard patient care order to address common hospital complaints such as nausea and therefore not having to write the order each time the patient becomes nauseous.

40. Imaging orders usually involve selecting a modality and specifying the region of interest. When ordering plain radiographs, the view must be specified. Computed tomography and magnetic resonance imaging can be done with or without contrast material and must be specified. A brief pertinent history and questions to be answered must also be provided.

41. Verbal orders are given directly to the nursing staff, either in person or over the telephone. These orders are recorded by the nurses in the medical record and eventually require a physician's signature. Orders such as these are typically given when either the physician is unable to physically write the order or in cases of emergency when orders need to be followed immediately.

42. DNR/DNI is an abbreviation for "do not resuscitate, do not intubate" and refers to a patient's code status. A patient is considered to be *full code* if he or she would like everything possible to be done in a code situation. Each patient, on admission to a hospital, should be asked about his or her desires if a medical catastrophe requires the use of code with "heroic measures."

43. Many patients will be admitted to the hospital with a provisional diet of NPO (*nil per os,* Latin for "nothing orally"). Patients who are expected to undergo certain imaging/studies or anesthesia/surgery will often be NPO to minimize the risk of aspiration. Theoretically, this is the initial default diet of every patient in the hospital, unless a physician has ordered a specific diet.

44. Any information in the medical record must be reviewed by a licensed medical professional. In some institutions, medical students can write, or "scribe" notes for physicians, but they must acknowledge that a licensed physician has reviewed the content recorded in the note. The acknowledgement/addendum is typically found at the end of the medical note.

45. Rounds are a medical team's daily evaluation of each patient cared for on a clinical service. This includes an organized assessment of the patient's diagnoses and pathologic condition as well as a formulation of a management plan.

46. There are various types of rounds, and they can be very different from each other. There are work rounds, teaching rounds, table rounds, and grand rounds. The attending on each service will decide on a day-to-day basis which types of rounds will occur.

47. Grand rounds are usually once-weekly gatherings of everyone within a specialty, from faculty, residents, or visiting professors. During these sessions, particularly interesting patients or areas of departmental research are commonly presented. These sessions can be thought of as hospital-wide teaching rounds. Each patient presentation is developed with the intention of educating the audience on a clinical topic.

48. Interns are a valuable resource for medical students. Because of their relatively recent completion of medical school, they are able to remember what it was like to be a medical student. Thus, they can offer advice and guidance on the basis of these experiences.

49. As a medical student (and even as an intern), you will typically need to arrive before the start of rounds. All patients will need to pre-round. Initially, pre-rounding will take more time until the routine has become more natural. Generally, allow for at least 15 to 20 minutes per patient at first. Depending on the service, the amount of detail to be collected on pre-rounds will vary significantly. Surgical services typically require far less time for pre-rounding than medicine services.

50. Pre-rounding occurs before rounds and involves collecting patient information such as overnight events from overnight residents or nurses, preparing to present the patient in front of the team, and formulating a medical management plan.

51. A good patient presentation is organized and succinct and delivers all of the pertinent information necessary to make a decision about the plan for the day. Achieving excellence in presenting patients may take a lot of practice.

52. There are two basic kinds of presentations: full presentations and daily progress presentations. Usually the full presentation is a verbal iteration of the full medical history and physical examination and is used only for the initial presentation (e.g., the morning after a patient has been admitted). The daily progress presentation is then used for all subsequent days spent in the hospital. Within these two types of presentations, the details required will vary from attending to attending.

53. Vital signs are recorded on flowsheets. Vital signs are usually recorded by the nursing staff, but at times it is advisable to take a manual pulse and measure a blood pressure if the recorded values do not seem correct. Some institutions record the vital signs electronically as well.

54. Flowsheets are the location on which a patient's information is recorded by the nursing staff. They are essentially timelines, with each flowsheet spanning a period of 24 hours over which the patient has various measurements recorded, such as vital signs, inputs and outputs, and pain scores. Flowsheets are generally located next to the patient's room or may be recorded online if the hospital has an electronic medical record.

55. Carding systems are an effective method of keeping track of patient information while they are on the inpatient wards.

56. If pimped or asked a question on rounds by the attending, try to think things through and provide a reasonable answer. Avoid just saying you do not know. If a question is answered wrong, be sure to read up on that topic because it may come up again.

57. When requesting a consult, be sure to have prepared a summary of the patient's presentation and medical problems, a specific question for the consulting team, recent vital signs and current medications, current patient location, and a contact phone or pager number.

58. When placing a consult request for a pediatric patient, be sure to check whether there is a separate pediatric consult team.

59. To prepare for a day in the operating room review the patient's medical record, identify any pertinent history or physical examination findings, and perform background reading on the patient's medical condition and the procedure. Be sure to pay special attention to the relevant anatomy.

60. Before surgery, medical students should introduce themselves to the patient in the preoperative holding area. If time allows, perform a focused history and physical examination.

61. Always wear clean scrubs in the operating room. T-shirts should not be worn underneath scrub tops. Be sure to wear proper identification, a cap, eye goggles, a mask, and shoe covers before entering the operating room.

62. After one completes the surgical hand scrub, it is important to avoid coming into contact with nonsterile objects and contaminating oneself.

63. The sterile zone includes the hands, arms, and anterior torso from the nipple line to the waist. It is important to remember that one's facial mask, goggles, and entire back, including the gown, are not sterile and therefore should not be touched by either hand. Any portion of the patient that is draped is considered sterile to the level of the tabletop. Anything below the level of the tabletop is not sterile.

64. To properly hold suture scissors, place the ring finger and thumb through the loops of the suture scissors and use the index finger to stabilize the scissors. Always cut with the tips of the scissors. Medical students should never grab the suture scissors on their own. Instead, politely ask the circulator nurse for the scissors and when done place them down for the circulator nurse to pick up. Do not place the scissors back on the circulator's tray.

65. The Bovie is an electrocautery device used during surgery. It can be used to produce vessel coagulation as it cuts, significantly decreasing the amount of bleeding during surgery. When used in the CUT mode, it provides a continuous electrical current to help cut through fascia, but with a decreased ability to coagulate vessels. In the COAG mode, it uses an intermittent electrical current that provides more vessel coagulation but decreased ability to cut.

66. Medical students should become familiar with the two-handed tie and instrument tie. A square knot tie involves one loop in the final step of the tie compared with a surgeon's knot, which has two loops.

67. Basic suturing patterns include simple interrupted sutures, running sutures, vertical mattress sutures, and horizontal mattress sutures.

68. The surgical team usually rounds before the day's first operation. Because the schedule is usually full of operations, the team has less time to round than teams on other services. In addition, the number of patients on a surgical service is often comparable (if not greater) than the number on a medicine service, so the pace must be increased.

69. Patients seen in the surgery clinic can be broadly divided into two categories. On one hand, surgeons will see postoperative patients in the clinic to ensure that the patient is recovering from surgery appropriately. On the other hand, surgeons will also evaluate patients with a variety of medical conditions to determine whether the patient is a suitable surgical candidate and whether the patient will benefit from a surgical procedure.

70. The intensive care unit (ICU) is a specialized area of the hospital designated for patients who are critically ill and may require increased monitoring, hemodynamic support, or airway support. One of the major differences in the ICU is that the nurse-to-patient ratio is higher (usually 1:2). In addition, "intensivists," who can provide care for patients, are available.

71. Patient monitoring is increased in the ICU. On the general floor, patient vital signs may be checked by nurses every 2 to 6 hours. In the ICU, the frequency of monitoring by nurses can range from every hour to as often as every 15 minutes, depending on the severity of illness. All patients in the ICU are in a "monitored bed," usually meaning that they are constantly connected to an electrocardiogram, pulse oxygenation, and blood pressure cuff monitor.

72. For floor patients, the plan is most commonly presented in a problem-based manner. However, for patients in the ICU, the plan is usually recorded and presented by systems. Because of the increased complexity of condition of ICU patients, presenting patients in this manner helps ensure that all problems are addressed.

73. Many patients in ICUs require intubation so that a mechanical ventilator can control the patient's breathing. Although there are several different methods of ventilation, the most common approaches are assisted control (AC), synchronized intermittent mandatory ventilation (SIMV), and pressure support ventilation (PSV). One important tip is that respiratory therapists are quite familiar with these machines and their settings and are a great resource for students to learn from.

74. The word *code* is used in hospitals to refer to a patient who is in cardiopulmonary arrest. When a code occurs, the code team is paged to rush to the patient's side to begin immediate resuscitation efforts. All residents in the hospital are trained in advanced cardiac life support (ACLS).

75. If a patient is physically unable or not mentally competent to make proper decisions, physicians must determine whether the patient has created an advanced directive. An advanced directive is a document in which a patient states his or her wishes about future medical care if he or she becomes unable to communicate or make competent decisions. A durable power of attorney and a living will are types of advanced directives.

76. If the patient does not have an advanced directive, the family can be consulted to make medical decisions. If the family is unavailable, the physician may make decisions that are in the best interest of the patient's medical care.

77. The decision to discharge a patient from the hospital depends on resolving or stabilizing the acute medical issues that the patient originally presented with and the issues that may not be manageable in the outpatient setting.

78. Almost all hospitals require that a patient have a physical examination conducted by a physician on the day of discharge. A complete physical examination should be performed, paying special attention to any portions of the examination that are related to the patient's reason for hospital admission.

79. The majority of patients will be discharged to go home. However, some patients may require additional medical attention that cannot be provided at home. The patient can either go home and have a visiting nurse provide some aspects of home medical care or they may go to another facility (such as an extended care facility) for further care.

80. The discharge process can become very complex with the large number of tasks that must be accomplished before completion of patient discharge. Many larger institutions are now hiring a permanent staff member, referred to as the discharge coordinator, discharge planner, or discharge nurse, to facilitate many of the tasks needed to arrange for a patient to have a smooth transition out of the hospital.

81. Patient education, medications/prescriptions, and follow-up medical care visits are the main components of the discharge instructions.

82. Some of the more common reasons for delays in discharging a patient include pending laboratory and diagnostic tests, transportation, and waiting for beds to become available in extended care facilities.

83. Outpatient care is not appropriate if the patient is unstable and requires close monitoring or if subsequent treatment for the patient cannot be delivered at home (e.g., IV fluid or IV medications).

84. Primary care is the act of a healthcare provider that serves as the initial assessment of care for a patient. Primary care clinics are conducted in the outpatient setting and involve family physicians, internal medicine physicians, pediatricians, and some obstetrics/gynecology physicians.

85. All individuals should establish care in a primary care clinic. If possible, the clinic should be conveniently located and easily accessible.

86. The length of time of an outpatient visit depends on the reason for the evaluation. Yearly health maintenance examinations are usually scheduled for 45 minutes to 1 hour. Return visits for a chronic condition, such as diabetes, are usually scheduled for 15 minutes. New patient consultations at specialty clinics are usually scheduled for 30 or 60 minutes, depending on the clinic.

87. For an established patient in the outpatient setting, the history and physical examination should be focused on any changes from previous visits and any new complaints.

88. A health maintenance examination is typically conducted annually and involves an overall assessment of a patient's health history, medical risk factors, physical examination, and required laboratory or diagnostic testing. Appropriate patient education is also provided to encourage patients to be aware of their health status and methods for improvement.

89. If a patient is presenting in the outpatient clinic after recent discharge from the emergency department or hospital, it is important to review the discharge summary. Pay special attention to the reasons for the hospital visit, clinical course, discharge diagnosis, changes in medications, and existence of any unresolved issues.

90. A specialty clinic is for patients whose problems require the expertise of a specialist in a specific area of medicine such as cardiology or rheumatology.

91. Patients can be referred to a specialty clinic through several pathways, including from a primary care physician, from the emergency department, after discharge from the hospital, and from another specialty clinic.

92. Students should be as efficient as possible when presenting patients to staff in the outpatient setting because time is limited, and there are usually many patients scheduled for the clinic within one day.

93. The methods of medical documentation in the outpatient setting include handwritten notes and typed electronic notes. However, verbal dictation is also commonly used to make more efficient use of limited time.

94. When beginning a dictation state the name of the person dictating, name of the physician that cared for the patient, the patient's name, patient identification number, patient's date of birth, date of visit, and the type of clinic the patient was seen in.

95. All prescriptions should include the name of the patient, the date, the name of the medication, dispensing information, patient instructions, number of refills, the name of the physician, and a signature of the physician (his or her DEA number is also required for certain drugs).

96. The length of time before a patient should return for another outpatient visit depends on the reason the patient presented and the discretion of the physician. Health maintenance examinations typically are conducted annually. Acute issues often require little or no follow-up. Chronic medical conditions usually have regularly scheduled return visits.

97. Medical students will be expected to be able to perform a variety of procedures. Be sure to follow all standard barrier precautions and note that most procedures require proper supervision.

98. Geriatric functional assessment should include questions regarding the activities of daily living (ADLs) such as necessary assistance for bathing, dressing, toileting, transfers, grooming,

and feeding. It should also include questions regarding indirect activities of daily living (IADLs) such as necessary assistance for administering medications, obtaining groceries, preparing meals, driving and transportation, making a phone call, handling finances, housekeeping, and laundry.

99. Assessment of pediatric patients should include discussion regarding perinatal and neonatal information, nutrition habits and status, and developmental history.

100. If there is any unknown question regarding a patient's care on the wards, ask a physician for assistance.

CHAPTER 1

THE U.S. HEALTHCARE SYSTEM

Mitesh S. Patel

1. **List the major players within the U.S. healthcare system.**
   A general overview of the major players within the U.S. healthcare system is displayed in Table 1-1.

TABLE 1-1. THE MAJOR PLAYERS OF THE U.S. HEALTHCARE SYSTEM

Providers	Hospitals, physicians, nursing homes and home health, pharmacists, public health organizations
Payers/insurers	Government (Medicare, Medicaid, Veteran Affairs), managed care, employers, individual out-of-pocket (private, health maintenance organization, preferred provider organization, and others)
Suppliers	Pharmaceutical companies, medical device companies, biotechnology companies, medical equipment suppliers

2. **Define the role of a provider.**
   Any organization or person licensed to deliver medical care services.

3. **What is the distinction between payers and insurers?**
   A payer is any organization, group, or person that pays for the expenses associated with medical illness or injury of an enrollee or member. An insurer is an organization that allows multiple payers to pool risk over a larger group, and thereby each incurs a smaller fee to protect against a catastrophic medical event. Managed care, health maintenance organizations, and preferred provider organizations are insurers. Some organizations, such as Medicare, Medicaid, and Veteran Affairs, are insurers who provide payment through the U.S. Government.

4. **Define the role of a supplier.**
   Any organization or group that manufactures and/or develops a product or technique used for medical care.

5. **When was the first hospital established in the United States?**
   In 1751, Benjamin Franklin and Dr. Thomas Bond established the first hospital in the United States, located in Philadelphia, Pennsylvania.

6. **Describe the organizational management of a typical hospital.**
   Hospitals are typically managed by two distinct entities: (1) the hospital administration and (2) clinical medical staff. The Chief Executive Officer (CEO) of the hospital oversees all administrative and clinical operations. Hospital administration is organized by an executive committee and/or board of trustees, which govern the hospital's finance, building and grounds,

and public relations committees. The administrative division may also oversee the medical records department, security system, and other departments responsible for the daily operating functions of the hospital. In contrast, the medical staff (which may include the dean of the hospital's affiliated medical school) governs the clinical departments such as pediatrics, radiology, and urology. The department chairs are responsible for managing the structure and function of their respective departments, as well as the physicians within those departments. The nursing staff may governed by both the medical staff and the hospital administration. Because of the duality of power within a hospital system between clinical and administrative controls, it is not unusual for the CEO of the hospital to lack complete governing authority over the physicians within the same hospital.

7. **Describe the differences between a community hospital and a specialized hospital.**
A community hospital is typically considered to be an institution that provides general medical care in the primary and acute setting to meet the needs of the community's local people. A specialized hospital focuses on one or more medical specialties and does not always provide general medical care. Examples of specialized hospitals include psychiatric hospitals, children's hospitals, and orthopedic surgical hospitals.

8. **Describe the differences between nonprofit and for-profit hospitals.**
Whereas both nonprofit and for-profit hospital systems provide similar medical services, they maintain different financial management structures. Nonprofit hospitals are organized as nonprofit corporations, meaning they are not owned by private investors and are not responsible to any shareholders. It is important to note that this does not mean these hospitals do not realize profits but rather that they do not act to maximize profits for any group of shareholders. These hospitals are usually limited to producing only a certain percentage of profit per year, such as 3–4%. All other profits must be either reinvested into the hospital for further development of the hospital system or externally invested for capital gains, which can lead to greater hospital improvements in the future. This is the reason that many nonprofit research medical centers continue to renovate and build new hospitals and research departments. Although the corporation itself is limited in its ability to produce profits, the physicians and staff within the hospital are still able to produce a profit in return for their services.
For-profit hospitals are owned by shareholders who keep stock in the corporation. A for-profit organization is first and foremost responsible to its shareholders. The underlying goal is to maximize profits for its investors, which are the shareholders. Although these hospitals often provide excellent medical care, some may focus their care toward specialties that produce larger profits such as cardiology and provide fewer resources for less profitable departments such as emergency medicine. A few of the large for-profit hospital systems in the United States include Columbia/HCA, Tenet, and HealthSouth.

9. **Explain the role of a teaching hospital.**
A teaching hospital's mission is to provide medical training for residents and medical students, although not all provide training for both. The majority of teaching hospitals are affiliated with academic medical centers.

10. **Describe the role of a physician within an academic medical center.**
Physicians within academic medical centers may have several different roles encompassing patient care, teaching, research, and administrative duties. The amount of time spent between these various roles differs by physician. In non-academic hospitals, physicians may still split time between these roles. However, physicians in non-academic hospitals are more likely to focus a majority of their time on patient care. In contrast, it is not uncommon for academic physicians to see patients 1 or 2 days per week and then spend the rest of their time teaching and/or conducting research.

11. What is the role of JCAHO?

JCAHO stands for the Joint Commission on Accreditation of Healthcare Organizations. JCAHO is responsible for setting the minimum standards of healthcare for all U.S. hospitals. Throughout the year, the organization visits each hospital to ensure that these standards are maintained and accreditation is justified. JCAHO is now more commonly known as The Joint Commission.

12. What is a hospital information system?

It is a complex, integrated system designed to optimize storage and transfer of information for both administrative and clinical divisions of the hospital. This system can be electronic and/or paper and may involve the use of one or more software programs. More recently, hospitals have been moving toward becoming paperless through the implementation of the electronic medical record (EMR) and computerized physician online electronic (CPOE) ordering system.

13. What is the role of health insurance?

The purpose of health insurance is to pool risk and protect one from incurring a substantial financial loss related to a medical expense.

14. Describe the Medicare program.

Medicare is a federally funded insurance program that provides coverage mainly to patients aged 65 years or older. The program was implemented in 1965 as an addendum to the Social Security Act. It was later expanded to cover blind individuals, patients with end-stage kidney failure, and younger disabled persons. Persons age 65 and older are automatically enrolled in Medicare Parts A and B if they have paid Social Security payroll taxes for a minimum of 10 years while employed, or if they meet other specific requirements. Patients with Medicare must still pay a monthly fee that is subsidized by the government and therefore relatively less expensive than most private insurance premiums. Many people may additionally still have copayments, deductibles, or other healthcare costs. The amount depends on the insurance plan they choose to enroll in.

The Medicare program is currently split into several parts. Part A is responsible for hospital reimbursement. Part B provides physician reimbursement. Medicare+Choice, sometimes referred to as Part C, includes healthcare plans that must be obtained through private insurance and requires participation in Parts A and B. Medigap is a plan sold through private insurance companies to fill the gaps in Parts A and B. Part D was implemented with the passage of the Medicare Prescription Drug, Improvement, and Modernization Act of 2003. The purpose of Part D was to provide some drug prescription coverage. However, the coverage can vary significantly from state to state.

15. Describe the Medicaid program.

Medicaid is both a federal and state funded insurance program that provides coverage mainly to the poor, as defined by those individuals maintaining a certain income level relative to the federal poverty line. It also provides a significant amount of coverage to children and pregnant women living at certain thresholds of the poverty level. The program was implemented in 1965 along with Medicare as an addendum to the Social Security Act. Although it is a federal program, money is divided among each of the states and is used as dictated by each state's legislation. Therefore, there is state-by-state variation in eligibility specifications and insurance benefits.

16. List the federally owned health systems.

Currently there are three federally owned health systems: the Veterans Health Administration, the Department of Defense, and the Indian Health Service. Hospital care clinic visits and insurance are included in these health systems. These health systems are distinctly different from nonprofit and for-profit health systems.

17. **Describe the role of the Veterans Health Administration.**
The Veteran Affairs (VA) health system is a federally funded organization run by the Veterans Health Administration that provides eligible veterans with hospital and clinic care, as well as insurance coverage, all within its own organization. About 5–6 million patients receive care through the VA health system. More than 20 million patients are eligible for coverage, but many choose to receive care elsewhere. The amount of coverage can vary and is dependent on time served in the military, setting of military service, and service-related disability. Prescription drug coverage is available to some patients, although there may be an associated copayment. VA hospitals are unique in that they do not have a level 1 trauma emergency department. Many patients receive initial care at larger hospitals and then are transferred to the VA hospital after their condition is stabilized. About two thirds of VA hospitals are set up in close proximity to academic medical centers and are staffed by academic physicians.

18. **How do medical records in the VA health system differ from those of other systems?**
The VA health system has the United States' only nationalized electronic medical record called the Computerized Patient Record System (CPRS). A patient can receive care in a VA hospital in California on one day and then go to a VA hospital in New York a day later and have all medical records available. Although the VA health system has offered to provide CPRS to other health systems at no cost, thus far nobody has begun using it. The main reason is that CPRS does not have a billing system linked to its medical records. Although this type of system works for the government-funded VA health system, others cannot implement an electronic system without a billing component.

19. **Describe the role of the Department of Defense in health care.**
TRICARE is a regionally managed healthcare program run by the Department of Defense to provide healthcare services for military personnel, military retirees, and their dependents. Healthcare is also provided for the direct families of these members.

20. **Describe the role of the Indian Health Service.**
The Indian Health Service is responsible for providing federal health services to American Indians and Alaska natives.

21. **What is managed care and how did its role develop in the United States?**
Managed care is a system originally designed to control the cost of care while trying to maintain the quality of care and patient satisfaction. The concept was first promoted by the Nixon Administration under the direction of Dr. Paul Elwood in the 1960s. In 1973, under the Reagan Administration, the Health Maintenance Act was passed as the first form of managed care. Managed care has been credited with controlling some of the rising cost of medical care in the 1980s and again in the 1990s under the Clinton Health Plan. However, in the late 1990s, a managed care backlash ensued from patient and advocacy groups complaining that cost-control measures had gone too far. Although managed care has lost some popularity, it is estimated that almost all facets of healthcare have some remnant of managed care influence.

22. **What is a health maintenance organization (HMO)?**
An HMO is a system designed to produce cost savings by creating an optimal protocol system. HMOs contract their own physicians and staff. Primary care physicians (PCPs) serve as gatekeepers to specialized care and are typically required to follow several protocols for a variety of processes including diagnostic tests and choice of prescription medications. Patients are commonly required to provide a copayment for each visit to their PCP. Additionally, they are limited to visiting only the physicians within the HMO network.

23. **Explain how a preferred provider organization (PPO) differs from an HMO.**
Although PPOs form contracts with physicians who will provide services, they allow patients to visit physicians outside of the network in return for a payment premium. Additionally, PPOs generally do not have copayments and instead offer deductibles and coinsurance programs.

24. What are out-of-pocket costs?
These are costs that are directly covered by the patient. There are three common types of out-of-pocket expenses that may be incurred while the patient has insurance. These three costs and their descriptions are displayed in Table 1-2. These costs may occur independently or simultaneously.

TABLE 1-2. TYPES OF OUT-OF-POCKET COSTS

Deductible	An amount the patient must pay for healthcare before the insurance will begin to cover expenses
Copayment	A fixed sum of money that is paid by the patient at the time of service from the provider
Coinsurance	A proportion of total healthcare costs that must be paid by the patient for all medical care related expenses

25. What is the role of a pharmaceutical company?
Also known as drug companies, these businesses focus on research, development, marketing, and sales of medical drugs for the healthcare industry.

26. What is the main cost driver for pharmaceutical companies?
Drug discovery and development comprise the most significant portion of cost for these companies. Drugs must pass through preclinical and clinical trials before receiving approval from the Food and Drug Administration (FDA) to ensure product safety and efficacy. Only a very small proportion of developed drugs survive the rigorous approval process.

27. What are drug patents and how do pharmaceutical companies benefit from them?
Because of the high cost of research and development, pharmaceutical companies require some incentive to continue producing drugs. Patents are this incentive. A patent duration varies but can last up to 20 years. The life of a patent begins at the time of patent filing, usually long before clinical trials take place. After a drug receives approval, there may be only a few years left on the life of the patent. During that period, others are restricted from producing the same product, and therefore the drug can be sold at a higher price because of a lack of competition. Once a patent expires, competitors can enter the market and the price of the drug will usually drop significantly after generics are introduced. There are a variety of circumstances under which a patent's life can be extended. However, these apply to only a small portion of all patents.

28. What is a biotechnology company?
Biotechnology companies leverage their technological application of biological systems and/or living organisms to create products and/or processes for a specific use. The two largest revenue-producing biotechnology companies in the United States are Amgen and Genentech. One of Amgen's top selling drugs is Enbrel (etanercept), a tumor necrosis factor-α (TNF-α) receptor blocker used to help decrease the symptoms of autoimmune illnesses such as rheumatoid arthritis, ankylosing spondylitis, and psoriasis.

29. What are differences between pharmaceutical companies and biotechnology companies?
Historically these two company types were more differentiated, but now they are very similar. Pharmaceutical companies classically discovered and developed small molecule compound

therapeutics, whereas biotechnology companies discovered and developed biological therapeutics such as recombinant proteins and gene therapy. As each of these industries has adopted some of the other's techniques, the differences have become less clear. Many have begun to describe both of these collectively as the pharmaceutical industry. Recently, pharmaceutical companies have even functioned under the same parent company.

KEY POINTS: THE U.S. HEALTHCARE SYSTEM

1. The major players in the U.S. healthcare system can be divided into the providers, payers/insurers, and suppliers.
2. The organizational management of a typical hospital is divided into two entities: the hospital administration and the clinical medical staff.
3. The purpose of health insurance is to pool risk and protect one from incurring a substantial financial loss related to a medical expense.
4. Medicare and Medicaid are federally funded insurance programs for particular subsets of the U.S. population.
5. In the past pharmaceutical and biotechnology companies were very distinct; however, now they are becoming very similar and occasionally function under the same parent company.

CHAPTER 2

THE EMERGENCY DEPARTMENT

Aditi Saxena

1. **What is the purpose of the emergency department (ED)?**
   The purpose of the ED is primarily to stabilize the patient, provide a diagnosis if possible, initiate treatment, and determine patient disposition. Possible dispositions include discharge to home, admission to an inpatient floor, or temporary observation.

2. **Describe the law regarding the ED's responsibility for patient treatment and transfer.**
   The Emergency Medical Treatment and Active Labor Act (EMTALA) was a statute passed in 1986 as part of the Consolidated Omnibus Budget Reconciliation Act (COBRA). This law requires that any patient who comes to the ED requesting examination or treatment for a medical condition must be provided with an appropriate medical screening examination, and, if determined to have an emergency condition, must be treated until stable regardless of ability to pay. Under this law, the hospital must also be sure to properly stabilize the patient before considering transfer to another facility.

3. **List the staff in the ED and describe their roles.**
   There are various physicians, physician extenders, nurses, and staff within the emergency department. Their roles are described in Table 2-1.

TABLE 2-1. ROLES OF THE EMERGENCY DEPARTMENT (ED) STAFF

Staff	Role
ED physicians	Provide medical care including patient assessment, treatment, and disposition. Can include attending physicians, emergency medicine residents, and off-service residents.
Off-service residents	Residents training in other specialties may rotate in the ED to gain experience with emergency care. In addition to providing care, they may also have specific roles varying by institution, such as determining to which inpatient service a patient should be admitted.
Physician extenders (e.g., physician assistants)	Healthcare professionals with specific postgraduate training. Depending on state laws, they may be able to practice independently, although most operate under the direction of a physician.
Nurses	Conduct regular checks on the patient, check vital signs, administer medications, and execute physician orders. In some situations, they may be able to initiate orders on specific patients (e.g., ordering x-rays on a patient with a wrist injury).

(Continued)

TABLE 2-1. ROLES OF THE EMERGENCY DEPARTMENT (ED) STAFF (CONTINUED)

Staff	Role
Technicians (e.g., emergency medical technicians or paramedics)	May start intravenous lines and draw blood samples. Depending on their level of training, they may also be able to apply splints or perform electrocardiograms. However, they cannot write prescriptions.
Clerks	Manage phone calls and paging, submitting orders, general paperwork, and patient registration. May also serve roles as patient liaisons.
Social workers	Arrange outpatient needs for patients who are uninsured, have limited access, or have other extenuating circumstances.
Trauma team	A team of surgeons, residents, physician extenders, and nurses that is responsible for patient care during a trauma situation along with the ED staff. Although this team is not actually a part of the ED staff, they are on call in larger institutions and are usually in the ED before patient arrival.
Consultants	Provide a specialist opinion when ED physicians feel it is necessary for patient care.

4. **Describe the layout of the ED.**
In general, most EDs consist of a waiting room, triage area, patient rooms, trauma/resuscitation bays, an urgent/minor emergency area, and an observation area.

Patient rooms are usually standardized across an individual ED. When one starts an emergency medicine rotation, it is a good idea to look through a patient room to learn what is available and where things are located. Many hospitals will have set locations in the hallway for patients when other patient rooms become full. These locations are surrounded by curtains and are commonly referred by a numbering system for the hallways within the ED. Some hospitals will have additional rooms for specific injuries such as an ophthalmic room with a portable slit lamp for patients with acute eye injuries.

The trauma/resuscitation bays are reserved for patients with the most severe injuries. These bays are larger in area, allowing more room for the multiple healthcare providers involved in patient care. They are equipped with additional materials, such as surgical lighting, telemetry, a portable ultrasound machine, and quick access to other portable radiology machines.

The urgent/minor emergency area is for patients who do not require extensive work-up, such as patients with simple lacerations that need suturing. This area usually has limited space and less equipment.

The observation area is generally reserved for patients who are awaiting admission to the floors or who are being followed as part of a protocol but no longer require active management. For example, patients with chest pain, who are deemed to have low-risk for myocardial infarction (MI) after an initial work-up, might be followed with serial cardiac enzyme measurements in an observation area as part of a "chest pain protocol."

5. **List the possible patient pathways into the ED.**
Patients can enter the ED through a variety of mechanisms. Upon arrival they enter triage and are subsequently sent to the appropriate location within the ED. The various pathways through which patients may arrive are displayed in Fig. 2-1.

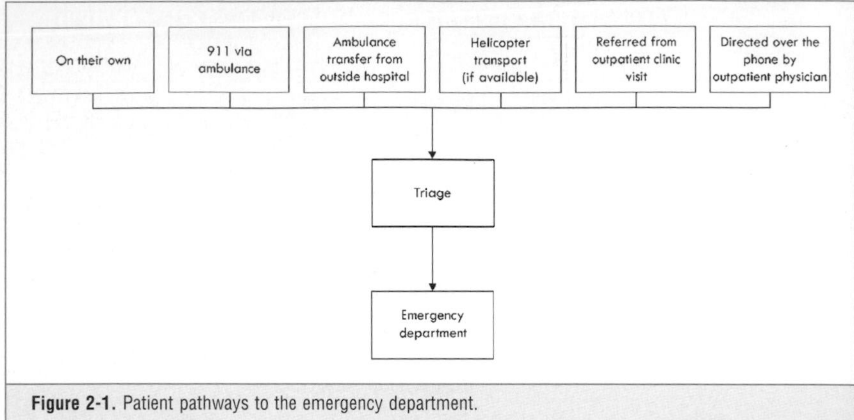

Figure 2-1. Patient pathways to the emergency department.

6. **What is triage?**
When patients arrive at the ED, they are first sent to triage. The process of triaging includes obtaining a patient's vital signs including temperature, heart rate, blood pressure, respiratory rate, and oxygen saturation, along with a brief history of the reason for presentation. Most patients are assigned a priority level on the basis of their vital signs and the severity of their condition. The patients with the most acute conditions, such as those with chest pain or difficulty breathing, are taken to a treatment room immediately and are seen by a physician as soon as possible. Patients who appear stable with less acute complaints may be initially sent to the waiting room, depending on the availability of patient rooms. If patients require immediate resuscitation, such as for respiratory distress, active seizure, or severe trauma, they may bypass triage and be taken directly to the trauma/resuscitation bay for initiation of care.

7. **What is a medical student's role during the emergency medicine rotation?**
The medical student's role primarily includes the following: gathering a thorough history, performing a full physical examination, presenting pertinent positive and negative symptoms to either a resident or attending physician, proposing a differential diagnosis, and suggesting follow-up laboratory results and studies. Before beginning to gather a history, be sure to quickly check the patient's vital signs and to ensure that the patient is stable. If the patient appears unstable, find a resident or attending physician immediately to determine whether immediate action is necessary before obtaining a history. Please note that time in the ED is limited. A general guideline is for students to try to conduct their assessment in 30 minutes, with 15 minutes to obtain the history, 10 minutes to conduct the physical examination, and 5 minutes to organize thoughts and devise a plan.
Medical students are also involved in performing a variety of procedures, such as starting intravenous lines (IVs), placing Foley catheters, placing nasogastric (NG) tubes, and drawing blood for measurement of arterial blood gases (ABGs). Under supervision, students may also participate in lumber punctures, central line placement, chest tube insertion, and endotracheal intubation.

8. **How should a patient presentation in the ED be structured compared with a similar presentation on the inpatient wards?**
Compared with the inpatient environment, time is limited and interruptions are frequent in the ED. A presentation of the history should include a one- to two-sentence synopsis at the beginning of the presentation followed by further details. Focus on pertinent positive and negative symptoms. When presenting the physical examination, be sure to include vital signs such as temperature, heart rate, blood pressure, respiratory rate, and pulse oximetry. These tend to play a crucial role in the ED and should not merely be summarized as "vital signs stable."

Presentation of the physical examination should include only relevant information. After the physical examination, continue with pertinent laboratory results and studies performed recently. When presenting a differential diagnosis, be sure to include a broad range of possibilities. Include anything that could severely harm the patient, and consider these possibilities first! Remember to think about multiple organ systems and to not just focus on the obvious one. Some students find it helpful to think of two parallel (and sometimes overlapping) differential diagnoses, one of which considers the life-threatening conditions of a symptom and another that consists of the most common. Next, present supporting and refuting information for each diagnosis in the differential. Finally, propose a plan for further laboratory results and studies to determine what steps are necessary to stabilize the patient or narrow the differential diagnosis.

9. **Explain shift work.**
   In the ED, faculty and staff work in shifts. Common shift lengths are 8, 10, or 12 hours. An example of a shift schedule would be a day shift from 7 AM to 3 PM, an evening shift from 3 PM to 11 PM, and a night shift from 11 PM to 7 AM. Shift changes are generally staggered among attending physicians, residents, and nurses to provide some continuity of care and to ensure that all staff taking care of one patient do not switch at the same time. Because new attending physicians and residents come on every shift, there is no overnight call. Instead, there are shifts during the night.

10. **How is shift work different than an inpatient schedule?**
    When "on service" in an inpatient service, medical students and residents are expected to stay until all work for that day for all patients on the service is complete. At that time, residents sign out their patients to the residents on call. Unlike the traditional inpatient schedule, when working in the ED, medical students and residents finish at the end of their shift. Different medical students and residents start with the next shift. At each shift change, the physician finishing up will sign out all of the patients he or she has been following to the physician coming on. Sign out involves a careful transfer of patient care to the oncoming team, including a review of the medical history, description of pertinent physical examination findings, a synopsis of laboratory results and studies performed thus far, a list of further necessary laboratory results, studies, and consults, and a presumed disposition. Conscientious transfer of care is essential for patient safety and high-quality care.

11. **How many shifts do emergency medicine physicians work?**
    Emergency medicine physicians typically work 12–16 shifts per month. These shifts are usually divided among day, afternoon, and night shifts. Some physicians may work fewer shifts because of administrative or research commitments. ED physicians often have the ability to make scheduling requests to accommodate personal obligations. In addition, some hospitals will "weigh" shifts differently. For example, a day shift might be worth 0.8 shifts, an evening shift worth 1.0 shift, and a night shift worth 1.2 shifts. Medical students are usually required to work 12–15 shifts during an emergency medicine rotation, but this varies by institution.

12. **How are emergency medicine physicians paid?**
    Physician reimbursement for medical services within the emergency department varies by institution and sometimes even within a single hospital. Physicians are most commonly paid either with an annual salary or by the hour. Some hospitals will pay physicians more during the night to encourage physicians to work these shifts.

13. **Describe how ambulance vehicles are positioned for anticipated emergencies.**
    Because emergencies are not scheduled occurrences, it is often difficult to anticipate the location of a future incident. However, certain locations such as urban areas typically have more emergencies than rural towns and are therefore covered by more

ambulance vehicles. One common technique is as follows. Within a specific area, several ambulances are positioned so that they are equidistant to all locations in the area. When an ambulance is called in for an emergency, the remaining vehicles must be repositioned so that they are again equidistant. Because of this technique, an ambulance vehicle may move many times throughout the night despite not being called in to provide medical care.

14. What is the role of the medical student while in an ambulance?

Some institutions allow medical students to take shifts in an ambulance usually in an observer capacity. When arriving to an emergency, students must be sure to first survey the scene to assure it is safe to enter. This involves taking cues from the more-experienced medics and avoiding placing oneself in jeopardy such as in the flow of traffic or becoming exposed if there is ongoing gunfire or interpersonal violence. Once on the scene, a medical student may be allowed to do a number of tasks under supervision of the medics such as obtaining a history, performing chest compressions, intubating, or placing an intravenous line. The other members of the ambulance team will facilitate what the student can and cannot perform. Students should take advantage of the medics' experiences and learn about prehospital care issues. In addition, a student may be able to provide additional education about more detailed medical concepts.

15. What are the ABCs?

In the emergency department, people will often refer to the *ABCs*. The ABCs stand for **A**irway, **B**reathing, and **C**irculation. It is important to first assess these three factors in the initial examination of a patient. In the ED, while assessing the airway, also be sure to protect the cervical spine if there is any concern regarding trauma.

Another common mnemonic used in the ED is *ABC-IV-O2-Monitor*. This refers to assessing the ABCs, then inserting necessary intravenous lines, providing the patient with oxygenated air for breathing, and attaching a cardiac monitor.

16. Describe the approach to a trauma patient.

The approach to a trauma patient is defined by advanced trauma life support (ATLS), which is a product of the American College of Surgeons. This approach is taught in a 2-day course, which is summarized briefly in Table 2-2. Most medical centers will also have a trauma system that activates both the ED and a surgical team to jointly and expeditiously evaluate patients with potentially serious injuries.

TABLE 2-2. APPROACH TO TRAUMA PATIENT

Airway	Assess airway and provide support (i.e., supplemental oxygen or endotracheal intubation) as indicated. Avoid manipulation of cervical spine.
Breathing	Listen to breath sounds bilaterally. Evaluate for pneumothorax or impaired air exchange.
Circulation	Feel for a pulse. Look at blood pressure and heart rate. If unstable, evaluate for source of bleeding. Consider potential of internal bleeding.
Disability	Assess the patient using the Glasgow Coma Scale and evaluate for evidence of spinal cord injury (paraplegia or quadriplegia).
Exposure	Remove the patient's clothes and examine for injuries. Do not forget to inspect the back using a "log roll" technique.

(Continued)

TABLE 2-2. APPROACH TO TRAUMA PATIENT (CONTINUED)	
Rectal	Perform a rectal examination to evaluate for rectal tone as a marker of neurologic status.
Tubes	Place nasogastric tube and Foley catheter unless contraindicated.
Imaging	All trauma with significant mechanisms should have portable chest and pelvic x-rays as part of the initial assessment. If there is the potential for internal bleeding, a focused assessment with sonography in trauma (FAST) examination should also be performed.

17. **What are the contraindications to placing a Foley catheter?**
Foley catheter placement is contraindicated in patients with urethral injury. Blood at the urethral meatus, a scrotal hematoma, a displaced pelvic fracture, or a high-riding prostate gland on rectal examination should raise a high suspicion for urethral tear. Retrograde urethrography, a procedure in which contrast material is injected into the urethra and x-rays are taken to provide visualization, should be performed in these situations before placing a Foley catheter.

18. **What is FAST examination?**
FAST is an acronym for focused assessment with sonography in trauma. The FAST examination is performed with a portable ultrasound machine and is used to evaluate for intraperitoneal bleeding in trauma patients. It has now essentially replaced diagnostic peritoneal lavage as the initial test for intraperitoneal bleeding. Using the ultrasound probe, four views are examined as shown in Fig. 2-2. The right upper quadrant view evaluates for blood between the liver and kidney in Morrison's pouch. The subxiphoid view evaluates for blood between the heart and pericardium (pericardial effusion). The left upper quadrant view evaluates for blood between the spleen and kidney. Lastly, the bladder view evaluates for fluid in the pouch of Douglas, the space posterior to the bladder. The FAST examination can detect as little as 300 mL of free fluid. Observation of free intra-abdominal fluid in a hemodynamically unstable patient is considered an indication to take the patient directly to the operating room.

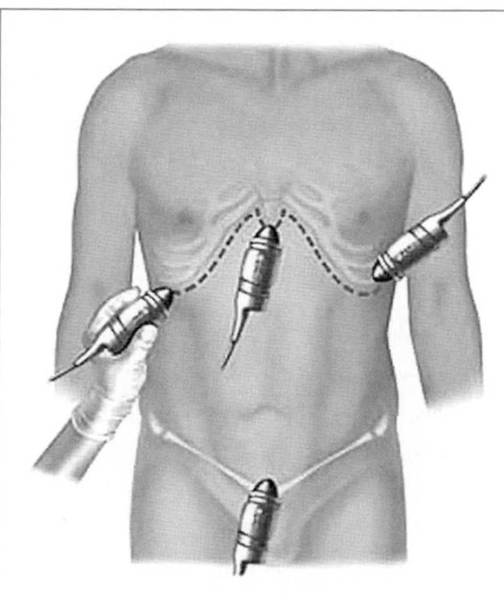

Figure 2-2. Four areas of evaluation using the focus assessment with sonography in trauma (FAST) examination. (From Rozycki GS, Feliciano DV, Schmidt JA, et al: The role of surgeon performed ultrasound in patients with possible cardiac wounds. Ann Surg 223:737, 1996, with permission.)

19. List the criteria to "clear" a cervical spine?

The National Emergency X-Radiology Utilization Study (NEXUS) group developed five criteria, which if met, indicate a low risk for cervical spine injury. These criteria are listed in Table 2-3. If all of these criteria are met, a cervical collar can be safely removed because there is little risk of cervical spine injury. The Canadian cervical spine (C-spine) rules also include low-risk mechanism and an ability to painlessly rotate the neck 45 degrees (N Engl J Med 349:2510-2518, 2003).

As a student, you should always check with your supervising physician before removing a patient's cervical collar because the potential consequences of inappropriate mobilization include inflicting an avoidable spinal cord injury.

TABLE 2-3. CRITERIA FOR CLEARING A CERVICAL SPINE
1. Normal level of alertness
2. No evidence of intoxication
3. Absence of painful distracting injury
4. Absence of midline cervical tenderness
5. Absence of focal neurologic deficit

20. Describe the different suture types and uses for each.

Sutures are differentiated on the basis of thickness, absorbable versus nonabsorbable, monofilament versus braided, and natural fiber versus artificial. In general, nonabsorbable, monofilament sutures (e.g., Ethilon or Prolene) are most suitable for surface wound closure. These result in the least scarring and lowest infection risk. Deep or buried sutures must be absorbable (e.g., Vicryl). Sometimes absorbable sutures (e.g., chromic gut) are used when suture removal is problematic, such as with small children who may require sedation. Sizes include 2.0 (usually pronounced "two-oh"), 3.0, 4.0, 5.0, 6.0, and 7.0. Suture size 2.0 is the thickest and is used for high tension surfaces such as the knee. A 5.0 or 6.0 suture is generally used for areas with less surface tension, such as the face. Natural fibers cause more inflammation than artificial fibers and therefore lead to increased scarring. As a result, they are used less frequently when cosmetic outcome is of concern. Silk is usually used for tying down lines and should never be used to close wounds because of the high infection risk and the high degree of scarring associated with it. Table 2-4 displays the different types of sutures, as well as their descriptions.

TABLE 2-4. DESCRIPTION AND COMMON USES FOR VARIOUS TYPES OF SUTURE

Suture Type	Description	Common Uses
Prolene	Synthetic, nonabsorbable, monofilament	Superficial wound closure
Ethilon	Synthetic, nonabsorbable, monofilament	Superficial wound closure
Vicryl	Synthetic, absorbable	Deep wound closure, intraoral suture
Silk	Natural, nonabsorbable	Tying down lines, never for wound closure
Chromic gut	Natural, absorbable	Used when removing sutures will be difficult

21. **What are other possible wound closure methods besides suture?**
Wound glue (Dermabond) and staples may also be used to close wounds. Staples are often used for linear lacerations and lacerations on the scalp. Please note not all wounds require closure. For example, puncture wounds from cat bites should not be closed because closure can increase the risk for infection.

22. **For burn patients, how is the percentage of body surface area burned determined?**
To approximate the percentage of a patient's surface area that is burned, use "the rule of 9 s." Each of the following equals approximately 9% of an adult patient's surface area: one arm, the anterior surface of one leg, the posterior surface of one leg, and the head. The chest and back each account for 18% of total body surface area. The genital region accounts for 1%. The hand itself is also considered 1%, and the size of the hand can be used to approximate smaller burns. These measures together with a measure for children (which is slightly different) are depicted in Fig. 2-3.

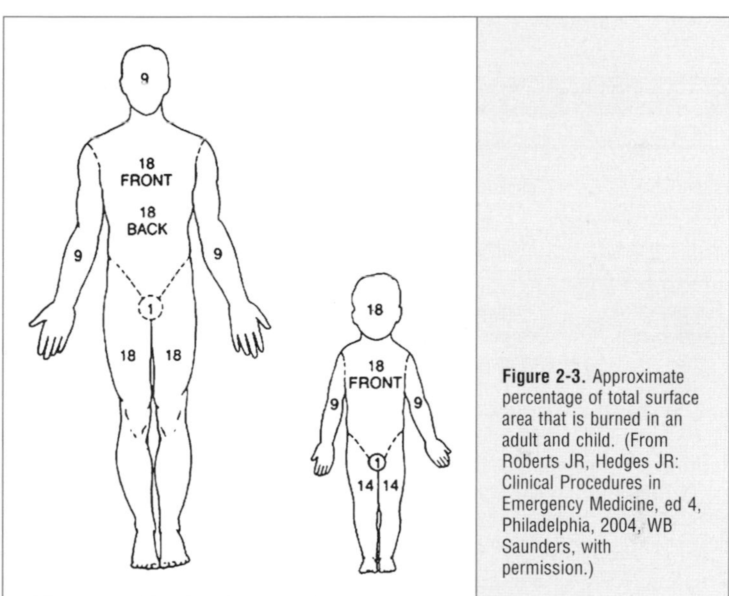

Figure 2-3. Approximate percentage of total surface area that is burned in an adult and child. (From Roberts JR, Hedges JR: Clinical Procedures in Emergency Medicine, ed 4, Philadelphia, 2004, WB Saunders, with permission.)

23. **List and describe the various types of burns. Provide examples.**
The four main types of burns are thermal, chemical, electrical, and radiation. Their descriptions along with examples are displayed in Table 2-5.

TABLE 2-5. TYPES OF BURNS

Type	Description	Example
Thermal	Burns due to contact with external heat source	Patient who burned herself with a curling iron
Chemical	Burns due to contact with strong acids or alkaloids	Pediatric patient who swallowed toilet bowel cleaner

(Continued)

TABLE 2-5. TYPES OF BURNS (CONTINUED)

Type	Description	Example
Electrical	Burns due to contact with an electric current	Patient who was struck by lightning
Radiation	Burns due to prolonged exposure to radiation	Patient who was sunburned due to ultraviolet radiation exposure

24. List and describe the classification system for burns. Describe the appearance of these burns.
Burns are described as either superficial, partial, or full thickness. They are often also described as first-, second-, or third-degree burns. The classification system, description, and skin appearance for each type of burn are outlined in Table 2-6.

TABLE 2-6. BURN CLASSIFICATION

Classification	Description	Skin appearance
Superficial (first degree)	Involves only epidermis.	Red, dry, no blisters, painful
Partial thickness (second degree)	Involves epidermis and part of dermis.	Red, blistered, painful
Full thickness (third degree)	Involves epidermis and entire dermis. May extend deeper to involve underlying tissues	Leathery, often with thrombosed capillaries; painless and burned area is minimally sensate

25. List reasons to refer a patient to a burn center.
Only certain larger hospitals contain a burn center. For minor burns, patients can usually be treated at any ED. However, several burn characteristics require patient referral to a burn center. These characteristics are displayed in Table 2-7.

TABLE 2-7. BURN CHARACTERISTICS REQUIRING REFERRAL TO BURN CENTER

1. 20% BSA burn on patients 10–50 years of age
2. Second- and third-degree burns >10% BSA on patients <10 or >50 years of age
3. Third-degree burns >5% BSA
4. Burns on face, hands, feet, eyes, genitals, perineum, or major joints
5. Circumferential burns on torso or extremities
6. High-voltage electrical burns
7. Inhalation burns
8. Significant chemical burns

BSA, Body surface area.

26. When is a specialty consult requested?

The decision to call for a consult is based on the discretion of the ED physician providing care for a patient. If the physician feels that the patient would benefit from the additional care and recommendations of a specialized physician, a consult is requested. There are some situations in which specialty consults are required, such as an orthopedic consultation for an open fracture.

27. Describe the possible patient dispositions.

Possible disposition for a patient seen in the ED includes going home, being admitted to an inpatient service, or being observed within the ED. If a patient is stabilized and his or her complaint has been treated, the physician might decide to discharge the patient and have him or her follow up with an outpatient physician if needed. When the physician's clinical judgment indicates that the patient requires medical care as an inpatient, the physician will choose to admit the patient to an inpatient service. Hospitals will have a variety of care levels available including general care beds (unmonitored), telemetry/monitored beds, stepdown units, and intensive care units. The ED physician in consultation with the admitting service must decide the appropriate level of care for each patient.

In other cases, patients are observed temporarily in the observation area until the decision to discharge or to admit is made at a later time, often on the basis of additional testing (e.g. cardiac stress test) or response to therapy (e.g. rehydration or asthma treatment).

28. What are observation protocols?

Patients who are stable and require additional treatment or evaluation, but are expected to be evaluated in less than 24 hours, may be moved to the observation area. These treatments and evaluations are commonly structured into protocols that require minimal physician intervention but still have clear, safe disposition. The most heavily studied type of ED observation protocol is for chest pain. A small percentage of patients with MIs have been inadvertently discharged from the ED, usually because of atypical presentations. To capture this group and identify patients at risk for MIs, chest pain protocols (CPCs) were developed. Patients receive serial cardiac enzyme testing, telemetry monitoring, cardiology consultation, and/or stress testing for rapid risk stratification. Observation protocols are also commonly used for patients with asthma, dehydration, cellulitis, transient ischemic attack, and atrial fibrillation.

29. What should be included in an ED discharge summary?

All discharge summaries from the ED should include a discharge diagnosis, discharge medications, and follow-up instructions. Thorough directions on medication administration should be provided in patient-friendly language. Follow-up instructions should include under what circumstances the patient should return to the ED. It is also important to outline when and where a patient should follow up in the outpatient setting. All of this information should be written legibly, reviewed with the patient, and acknowledged by the patient with a signature.

KEY POINTS: THE EMERGENCY DEPARTMENT

1. The purpose of the emergency department is primarily to stabilize the patient, provide a diagnosis if possible, initiate treatment, and determine patient disposition.
2. Under EMTALA all patients must receive proper medical screening and appropriate subsequent medical care regardless of ability to pay or lack of insurance.

3. Time is limited and interruptions are frequent in the emergency department, so the aim should be for all interactions to be concise and efficient.
4. Emergency medicine physicians typically work in shifts of set durations.
5. Disposition from the emergency department includes going home, inpatient admission, or observation.

THE ADMISSION PROCESS

Mitesh S. Patel

CHAPTER 3

1. **When does a patient get admitted to the hospital?**
   The decision to admit a patient for management and treatment within the hospital is based on clinical judgment, treatment protocols, and, most importantly, the patient's medical condition. Most of these decisions are made within the emergency department. Emergency medicine physicians are trained to resuscitate, diagnose, and plan disposition. The patient's disposition includes discharge, observation, or admission to the hospital. When the physician's clinical judgment determines that the patient requires care in an inpatient setting rather than an outpatient setting, the physician will choose to admit the patient.

   Certain patient presentations are identified by hospital protocol for admission. For example, almost all hospitals will admit a patient with active chest pain and electrocardiogram (ECG) changes, if not for treatment, then at least for monitoring of ECG rhythm, vital signs, and laboratory results.

2. **What if the patient does not want to be admitted?**
   In most situations, patients will agree to be admitted to the hospital. If the patient insists on leaving, the physician will typically clarify that medical advice warrants admission and document that the patient was informed of the medical recommendation but left against medical advice.

   There are several situations in which patients may be admitted against their will. When the patient expresses a plan to hurt himself or herself or others, he or she can be forced to be admitted to the hospital. When it has been determined that the patient does not have the mental capacity to make his or her own medical decisions, he or she can also be admitted without consent. When a patient arrives at the hospital in distress, needs emergency resuscitation or surgery, and is unable to give consent because of the presenting medical condition, the patient may be admitted without consent.

3. **From where are patients admitted?**
   Patients can be admitted to the hospital from several different settings as displayed in Fig. 3-1. The majority of patients are admitted from the emergency department. Once in the hospital, patients often move from one location to another (intra-/interservice transfer) based on the severity of their medical condition. An inpatient service may receive an admission from the operating room after surgery, from the intensive care unit (ICU) when the patient's condition improves, or from another inpatient service when one of several medical issues has resolved.

   For example, a patient in a motor vehicle accident might be taken straight to the operating room and then be admitted to the orthopedic surgery service for follow-up of a fracture repair (Surgery → Admit). This patient may then develop a pulmonary embolus and be transferred to the ICU for respiratory distress (Inpatient service → ICU). When the patient's status improves and breathing is done independently, he or she could be admitted to the general medicine service for continued care (ICU → Inpatient service). If the patient suddenly develops atrial fibrillation with an accelerated ventricular rate, he or she may need admission to the cardiology service (Inpatient service → Inpatient service). Although this situation is rare, it does occur and is an excellent example of the variability of patient admissions.

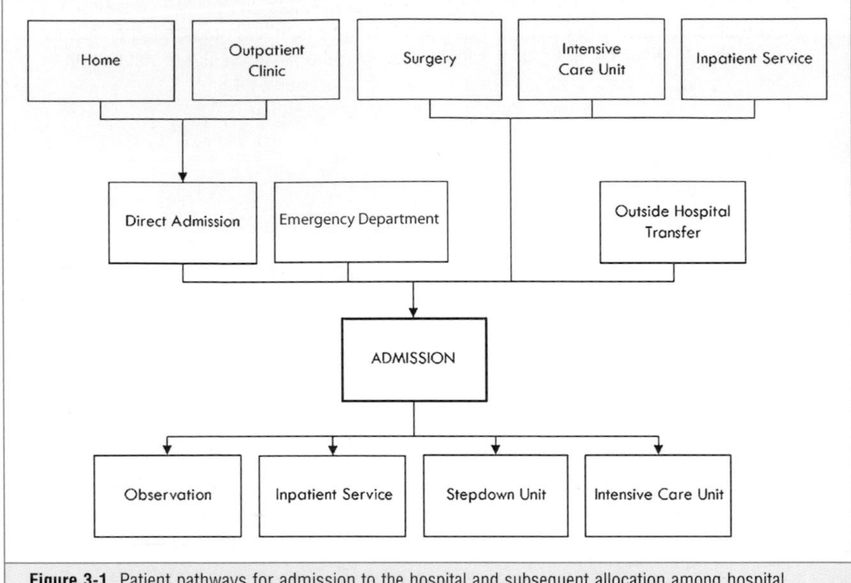

Figure 3-1. Patient pathways for admission to the hospital and subsequent allocation among hospital services.

Other possible sources for patient admissions include transfers from outside hospitals that do not have adequate resources or capabilities, direct admissions from outpatient clinics, and patients who called their physician for medical advice and were arranged for admission from home.

4. **To where are patients admitted?**
Most hospitals have two or more levels of inpatient care based on the severity of the patient's illness. Each level differs in the number of staff members per patient, frequency of care, and accessibility to extensive monitoring and treatment. Most hospitals have an observation unit (which may not be considered a hospital admission), an inpatient service with or without extensive monitoring, and an ICU. Some larger hospitals have levels of care between the ICU and inpatient service, commonly referred to as the *stepdown* unit.

5. **Who decides to what service a patient gets admitted?**
The majority of decisions as to which service to admit a patient to are controlled within the emergency department. In addition, a consulting service may choose to recommend admitting a patient to its service for further treatment. Some hospitals may have protocols for admitting procedures for "typical" patient presentations. For example, patients with chest pain may be sent to the cardiology service, whereas patients with seizures are sent to the neurology service.
When a patient is to be admitted to a general medicine service, there is often a resident within the emergency department who is assigned the role of allocating patients throughout the hospital. The allocation is dependent on severity of the patient's condition, distribution of patients within the hospital, and likely length of hospital stay. Each service may have a cap or quota—a maximum number of patients the service can accept each night. There are rules under which a service may have to accept additional patients above the cap

or quota. ICU patients commonly account for this. For example, the cardiology service may allow each of its interns to carry eight patients. Once this number is reached, the patients are admitted to the general medicine service. However, if a patient requires a stay in the coronary care unit, the service is required to take on that additional patient. There may also be services within various hospitals that do not have a cap or quota.

6. **What are the important portions of a history and physical examination that should be included during a patient admission?**

Every patient who is admitted to a service requires a complete history and physical examination, commonly known as the *Admit H&P.* Although the focus of this H&P will depend on the patient's presentation and the admitting service, the general outline in Table 3-1 can be followed to avoid leaving out important portions.

TABLE 3-1. ADMISSION HISTORY AND PHYSICAL EXAMINATION

Medical History		
Abbreviation	Name	Description
CC	Chief complaint	The patient's main problem requiring medical care.
HPI	History of present illness	A thorough description of the chief complaint and associated symptoms that have led up to the patient's current status. Include pertinent positives and negatives.
PMH/PSH	Past medical/surgical history	Any past medical conditions or surgeries related or not related to the chief complaint.
MEDS/ALL	Medications and allergies	All medications the patient is currently taking including dosages, as well as past or recent medications that are relevant to the HPI. Any over-the-counter (OTC) medications, herbal supplements, or vitamins. Any allergies the patient may have to medications or medical treatments.
FH	Family history	Any illnesses that may run in the family such as cancer, diabetes, or heart disease. Focus on illnesses that may be related to the chief complaint. Age and medical conditions of any siblings or children.
SH	Social history	Current location, living situation, marital status, and number of children; employment and education; tobacco, alcohol, or recreational drug use.

(Continued)

TABLE 3-1. ADMISSION HISTORY AND PHYSICAL EXAMINATION (CONTINUED)

Abbreviation	Name	Description
Medical History		
ROS	Review of systems/symptoms	Complete review of all patient symptoms within each of the organ systems.
CODE	Code status	Because the patient is in the hospital, it is important to determine whether he or she would like emergency resuscitation including intubation if necessary.
Physical Examination		
Abbreviation	**Name**	**Description**
VITALS	Vital signs	Includes temperature, heart rate, blood pressure, respiratory rate, and, if possible, oxygen saturation and/or oxygen requirement.
GEN	General	Description of patient's alertness and orientation (person, place, and time).
HEENT	Head, eyes, ears, neck, and throat	Full examination focusing on these anatomical areas.
CARDIO	Cardiovascular	Includes examination of heart, vessels (carotid arteries and internal jugular vein) and overall fluid status.
PULM	Pulmonary	Includes examination of lungs, upper airway, and chest wall.
ABD	Abdominal	Includes examination of gastrointestinal tract, liver, gallbladder, spleen, and abdominal wall.
SKIN/EXT	Skin and extremities	Full skin examination and color, warmth, and pulses of extremities.
GU/RECTAL	Genitourinary and rectal	Includes bladder, urinary tract, pelvic examination, and rectal examination. Medical students may require physician or staff supervision.
NEURO	Neurologic	Full neurologic assessment includes mental status, cranial nerves, motor (cerebellar function, muscle strength, and gait), reflexes, and sensation (proprioception, vibration, pinprink, and light touch).

7. List the components of the review of systems (ROS)?

A systematic approach is typically used to screen the patient for a range of symptoms that may be related to their history of present illness. Most hospitals require that at least 10 of 14 systems be reviewed to report accurate documentation and for billing purposes. Although no standard list exists, the systems and symptoms in Table 3-2 can be used as a guideline of the 14 systems. When asking patients about these symptoms, be sure to ask in patient-friendly terminology; for example, for paroxysmal nocturnal dyspnea, one could ask, "Do you ever wake up in the middle of the night short of breath?"

TABLE 3-2. REVIEW OF SYSTEMS

System	Symptoms
1. General	Fever, chills, night sweats, fatigue, sleep, change in weight
2. HEENT	Headaches, vision change, tearing, hearing change, nasal congestion or bleeding, ringing in ears, neck stiffness/soreness, lymphadenopathy, dental pain, mouth sores, sore throat
3. Chest/breast	Chest/breast masses, discharge, or pain
4. Cardiovascular	Chest pain, dyspnea on exertion, orthopnea, paroxysmal nocturnal dyspnea, edema, hypertension, murmurs, cyanosis, varicosities, phlebitis, claudication
5. Pulmonary	Cough, shortness of breath, sputum production, hemoptysis, wheezing, stridor, infections
6. Gastrointestinal	Nausea, vomiting, hematemesis, dysphagia, abdominal pain, diarrhea, constipation, melena, hematochezia, hemorrhoids, change in appetite or bowel habits, food intolerances, jaundice
7. Genitourinary	Urgency, frequency, hesitancy, dribbling, incontinence, dysuria, nocturia, hematuria, polyuria, oliguria, stones, infections, discharge, sexually transmitted diseases, irregular menstrual periods, excessive menstrual bleeding
8. Musculoskeletal	Joint pain, swelling, redness, muscle weakness, tenderness, cramps, range of motion
9. Dermatologic	Rash, itching, pigmentation, moisture or dryness, changes in hair growth or loss, nail changes
10. Neurologic	Seizures, vertigo, numbness, tingling, coordination difficulty, tremor, sensory disturbances, memory or speech problems
11. Psychiatric	Change in mood, depression, hallucinations, delusions, intent to hurt self or others
12. Endocrine	Heat or cold intolerance, excessive thirst, hunger, or urination
13. Hematologic	Anemia, abnormal bleeding, abnormal bruising, transfusions
14. Allergic	Asthma, hay fever, eczema, sinus problems

8. What should medical students do if the ROS list is not available?

Most students will not have Table 3-2 available to refer to while taking a history. If stuck and unable to remember what to ask next, try asking about general symptoms and then going from head to toe. An abbreviated example might be: "Do you have any fevers, chills, night sweats, change in weight/appetite? Do you have any headaches, changes in vision or hearing, runny nose or congestion, sore throat or cough, chest pain or shortness of breath, abdominal pain, nausea/vomiting, diarrhea/constipation, problems with urination or abnormal genitourinary discharge, muscle/joint aches, difficulty with walking or balance?" Other students may ask questions by thinking about each of the systems.

9. **List the steps involving in writing admission orders.**
Each patient admitted to a service needs a set of admission orders. These orders can usually be written by a medical student, but a physician must read over them and sign the orders. The staff is not allowed to carry out the orders until a physician has verified and signed them. A commonly used mnemonic to remember the steps of admission orders is ADC VAN DIMSL. Table 3-3 displays a list of possible options for writing admission orders.

TABLE 3-3. ADMISSIONS ORDERS

Admit to	List admitting service (i.e., cardiology, neurosurgery, general medicine). List admitting resident and attending with pager numbers.
Diagnosis	List the main diagnosis and any others that are related to patient care (i.e., chest pain, shortness of breath, vertigo).
Condition	Indicates severity of the patient's illness. Varies by hospital but examples are critical, guarded, fair, stable.
Vital signs	Indicates which vital signs should be taken and how frequently. Examples are q shift (q = every, a shift is typically 8 hours), q2 hours, q4 hours, etc. Many residents will write "per routine." You must know what this means at a particular hospital before you write it down.
Activity	Refers to limitations on activity. Examples include strict bed rest (do not get up), bed rest with bathroom privileges (only allowed to get up to use the restroom), up in chair bid (have sitting twice a day), ad lib (as tolerated), and no restrictions.
Nursing	Indicates care provided by nursing staff. Examples include daily weights (check weight every morning), strict Is & Os (record all intake and output), CR monitor (cardiorespiratory), and continuous pulse ox (oximeter).
Diet	Indicates what the patient is allowed to eat. Examples include NPO (nil per os = no eating or drinking), 1500 cal ADA (American Diabetic Association), low salt (patients with congestive heart failure), cardiac diet (a protocol diet at some hospitals), and no gluten (patients with celiac disease).
IV fluids	List the components of the fluid and the rate of intake. Examples include D5 1/2NS + 20 mEq/L KCl meaning 5% dextrose in ½ (or 0.45%) normal saline with potassium chloride.
Med/Allergies	List all the necessary medications. This may or may not include the medications the patient regularly takes at home. This will also include the new medications that are being started for treatment of the patient's diagnosis. Be sure to list any known patient drug allergies. If the patient has no allergies write NKDA (no known drug allergies).

(Continued)

TABLE 3-3. ADMISSIONS ORDERS (CONTINUED)

Special	List any diagnostic tests the patient may need. List any other special circumstances.
Labs	These should be the laboratory results you need now and the ones you want routinely. Be sure to determine whether the patient has already had some blood drawn (such as from the emergency department).

IV, Intravenous.

10. **What else should be written after ADC VAN DIMSL is completed?**
The house officer or resident taking care of this patient will write a set of orders indicating when the covering physician should be called or paged by staff. These orders usually cover minimum and maximum patient vital signs and other monitored values. The issues commonly include temperature, respiratory rate, oxygen saturation, heart rate, blood pressure, and urine output. Although the limits may need to be adjusted for each patient, for many patients the following order may be used: "Call HO if T >100.5, SBP >130 or <90, HR >120 or <60, RR >30 or <12, O2Sat <92%, UO <30 mL/hr" (HO = house officer). In addition, some patients will have additional monitoring with associated "Call HO" orders.

11. **How is the patient's past medical record related to the admission?**
Proper review of prior hospital admissions, recent outpatient notes, diagnostic tests, or laboratory results can help to formulate the course of the patient's illness. Many patients gradually progress toward the need for hospital admission. By reviewing this information before interviewing the patient, you can more properly focus your questions and physical examination. It is also important to note past physical examination findings such as murmurs or prior neuropathies so that you can assess whether a physical examination finding today is new or unchanged from the past. In addition, it is very helpful to the team if medical students review the past medical record for previous tests and studies, including previous ECGs, chest x-ray findings, echocardiogram results, or pulmonary function tests. Patients can be an excellent source of information to help describe or clarify their past medical history.

12. **If the patient has never been to this hospital, how are past medical records obtained?**
If the patient has previously received care at another health system, the medical records department at the other institution can be called and requested to send any existing records to the patient's current hospital. However, the patient's written consent must first be obtained to release these medical records. This form will typically need to be faxed to the hospital releasing the medical documentation. If the patient is not arousable or oriented enough to sign the form, the patient's legal guardian may be able to sign the release forms.

13. **Describe "staffing" the patient?**
Each patient admitted is usually first seen by a medical student or resident. After the Admit H&P has been completed, the medical student or resident must staff the patient with the attending physician who is responsible for the patient's care. This typically consists of a full presentation of the patient's history and physical examination, along with any pertinent laboratory results and studies. In addition, you will be required to give an assessment of the patient and a management plan. The attending physician will agree and disagree with various components of the presentation and will make all final decisions regarding the treatment plan.

14. **What should be included in your assessment of the patient?**
An assessment of the patient should be limited to a few lines of dialogue and should give a summary of the patient's age, gender, significant past medical history, significant risk factors, presenting signs and symptoms for this hospital admission, and differential diagnosis. The assessment is also sometimes referred to as the impression.

15. **Provide an example of a patient assessment.**
Mr. Smith is a 68-year-old man with a past medical history of hypertension, coronary artery disease, and chronic obstructive pulmonary disease presenting with two episodes of syncope over the past 24 hours probably due to atrial fibrillation versus transient ischemic attack.

16. **Describe the organization of the plan.**
There are two standard methods of organizing the management plan during a patient admission: a systems-based approach and a problem-based approach. The method that is chosen usually depends on the attending physician's or resident's preference. The plan can refer to any portion of the history and physical examination, laboratory results, or diagnostic tests that is part of the patient's admission.

17. **Explain a systems-based approach to the management plan and when it may be most beneficial.**
A systems-based approach is most effective for a patient with complex medical problems that involve multiple organ systems, such as patients in the ICU. Each system affected by the patient's medical condition should be addressed starting with the most important or most severe. Many physicians prefer that students use a systems-based approach in the beginning so that their assessment is complete and they do not leave anything out of the treatment plan.

18. **Explain a problem-based approach and when it may be most beneficial.**
A problem-based approach is most effective when the patient has only a few medical problems. Each problem should be listed, and all organ systems affected by that problem should be included in the plan. A problem-based approach can be dangerous because students may leave out important information that is not directly associated with one of the patient's main problems.

KEY POINTS: THE ADMISSION PROCESS

1. The decision to admit a patient for management and treatment within the hospital is based on clinical judgment, treatment protocols, and, most importantly, the patient's medical condition.
2. Patients can be forced to be admitted against their will if they express intent to harm themselves or others, or if they are judged to not have the mental capacity to make proper decisions.
3. Every patient who is admitted to a service requires a complete history and physical examination.
4. ADC VAN DIMSL is an excellent mnemonic for writing admission orders.
5. The two standard methods of formulating the management plan are a systems-based approach and a problem-based approach.

LABORATORY AND DIAGNOSTIC TESTS

Eric W. Schneider

1. **Describe the step-by-step process whereby laboratory results are obtained by the medical team.**
The first step in the process of obtaining laboratory results occurs when the medical team caring for the patient writes an order for a specific laboratory test. This can be either a paper order in the patient's chart or an electronic order through an online order entry system. A paper order is subsequently processed by the unit clerk who schedules the requested blood draw. The blood draw is generally performed by either the nursing staff or a dedicated phlebotomy team. The blood sample is collected in the appropriate tube and transported to the pathology and laboratory medicine department. The sample is then processed in the appropriate assay. At most institutions, the results are recorded online for medical staff to view, although certain hospitals continue to rely on paper copies of test results, which are kept in the patient's chart.

2. **Describe the process of blood sample collection.**
Blood samples are collected by some combination of dedicated phlebotomy teams, nurses, technicians, residents, and medical students. Most medical centers have phlebotomy teams whose chief responsibility is to make multiple rounds through the hospital to collect blood samples for ordered laboratory tests. For example, a phlebotomy team may be scheduled to conduct blood draws at 6:00 AM, 9:00 AM, 10:30 AM, 12:00 PM, 2:30 PM, 4:00 PM, and 9:00 PM. During the day, the phlebotomist retrieves laboratory requisitions from the floor clerk, identifies and confirms the correct patient, and proceeds to draw blood from the corresponding patient. The phlebotomist subsequently transports samples to the central distribution station, where it is then sent to the appropriate laboratory (e.g. hematology, chemistry, microbiology).

3. **What are A.M. labs?**
An important concept to be aware of in the blood sample collection process is that of *A.M. labs.* This term refers to specimens drawn during the first phlebotomy rounds of the day (such as 6:00 AM). Generally, A.M. labs consist of basic maintenance laboratory tests that are performed daily (or weekly depending on the particular test) and are written for during the preceding day. To illustrate this concept, consider a patient admitted with liver failure. A typical set of A.M. labs (i.e., daily maintenance laboratory tests) may consist of a comprehensive metabolic panel, coagulation tests (prothrombin time [PT], activated partial thromboplastin time [aPTT]), and a complete blood count (CBC). It is not uncommon for some residents to write for daily A.M. labs several days in advance. However, because the patient's medical condition is constantly changing, they must be careful to avoid ordering unnecessary tests or omitting required ones. When writing for A.M. labs, the abbreviation "AML" may be used. Make sure to include the date as well, for example: "AML 09/28: CBC, coags, etc."

4. **How are blood samples stored for transport to the pathology/laboratory medicine department?**
Samples are stored in tubes with special coatings. Each coating is represented by a different color tube top. The type of tube used for a particular blood sample is dictated by the intended

TABLE 4-1. COLOR-CODED BLOOD COLLECTION TUBE COATINGS AND ASSOCIATED COMMONLY ORDERED TESTS

Color	Coating	Commonly Ordered Tests
Red	None	For serum chemistry analysis (metabolic panels), blood banking (type and screen), and serologic tests (autoantibodies, viral antibody titers)
Gold	Gel separator with clot activator	For serum chemistry analysis (metabolic panels, liver function tests, cardiac enzymes, drug level monitoring, lipid panels)
Lavender, pink	EDTA	For whole blood assays (complete blood count [CBC], hormone levels)
Light blue	Sodium citrate	For coagulation assays (prothrombin time [PT], activated partial thromboplastin time [aPTT], clotting factor levels) on plasma or whole blood samples
Green	Sodium heparin	For plasma or whole blood chemistry analysis (metabolic panels, liver function tests, cardiac enzymes, drug monitoring, lipid panels)
Gray	Potassium oxalate/ sodium fluoride	For lactate, bicarbonate, glucose assays
Yellow	Acid citrate dextrose	Whole blood determinations including flow cytometry and tissue typing assays

laboratory test. The various colored tube tops, their coatings, and common tests for which they are used are listed in Table 4-1.

5. **Describe the difference between routine and STAT orders. How can the receipt of results from STAT be further hastened?**
The majority of laboratory requests written on patient care floors are *routine*. This means that necessary samples are drawn at regularly scheduled hours and processed in the order in which they are received in the pathology department. Although it varies widely depending on the volume of laboratory requests and type of test requested, routine results are usually available the same day (e.g., 4-6 hours for simple blood tests). Results that are required more urgently should be indicated as *STAT* requests. STAT requests generally have a much faster turn around time (e.g., $\approx$1 hour for simple blood tests). One may also speed the receipt of laboratory results by personally transporting specimens to the pathology/laboratory medicine department and by phoning the relevant laboratory within the department to request results, which avoids wait time related to posting results online.

6. **Which laboratory within the pathology/laboratory medicine department should be called to obtain a particular laboratory result?**
The pathology/laboratory medicine department is made up of several component laboratories that use distinctive assays to process different types of samples. To obtain an urgent result by phone or in person, you may want to try to contact the appropriate component laboratory. However, at most institutions if you call the central pathology laboratory, they can transfer you to the appropriate component. The common tests that may be performed by the various component laboratories are outlined in Table 4-2.

TABLE 4-2. PATHOLOGY LABORATORIES AND COMMONLY PERFORMED TESTS	
Chemistry	Metabolic panels, therapeutic drug monitoring, enzyme levels
Hematology	Complete blood count (CBC)/differential, peripheral smears, erythrocyte sedimentation rate (ESR)
Coagulation	Prothrombin time(PT); activated partial thromboplastin time (aPTT)
Microbiology/virology	Cultures, Gram stains, viral serologic tests, antibiotic sensitivities
Immunology	Autoantibodies, protein electrophoresis (urine/serum)
Histocompatibility	HLA typing
Blood bank	Type and screen

7. **Describe the process for retrospectively adding tests to a previously collected blood sample.**
Additional laboratory tests may need to be performed because of the discovery of new information regarding the patient's medical condition or because of the accidental omission of tests during order preparation. If this situation arises, be aware that the relevant laboratory within the pathology/laboratory medicine department (see Table 4-2) can be contacted to add on an omitted or newly desired assay after a specimen has already been collected. For example, additional electrolyte levels (such as magnesium or phosphorus) are often added on to a basic metabolic panel after a patient is presented during rounds. The ability of the laboratory to comply with your request depends on the amount of time that has passed since sample collection, the amount of sample remaining, and the type of tube in which the sample was collected. If this process is successful, additional blood draws are avoided. In addition, the results will typically be returned much faster than if another blood draw had to be done.

8. **When does a laboratory test need to be sent outside of the hospital to obtain results?**
Although most major medical centers have fairly comprehensive clinical laboratory facilities, certain specialized tests are "send outs." Send outs are assays that the institution does not have the capability to perform in-house and thus must be sent to another institution for processing. Results from such tests take much longer to receive (days or weeks rather than hours) owing to increased transport time as well as the specialized nature of the test. Examples of tests that are send outs at many hospitals are uncommon fungal or viral serologic tests (e.g., histoplasma antibody), autoantibody titers (e.g., acetylcholine receptor antibody), enzyme levels (e.g., arylsulfatase A), and hormone levels (e.g., glucagon).

9. **What are the two most common metabolic panels encountered on the wards? Compare and contrast their clinical use.**
The two most commonly used metabolic panels are the basic metabolic panel and the comprehensive metabolic panel. Both panels can be used to identify common electrolyte abnormalities as well as to monitor blood glucose and renal function. The comprehensive metabolic has the added benefit of providing information regarding transaminases, total bilirubin level, and total protein and albumin levels.

10. **List other common terms used to describe the basic metabolic panel?**
Synonyms for a basic metabolic panel include Chem-8 and SMA-8 (sequential multichannel analysis-8). The Chem-7, SMA-7/SMAC-7, and Metabolic Panel 7 are used at certain institutions.

They are identical to the basic metabolic panel with the exception of calcium, which is omitted. Certain institutions also use a Chem-4, which only assesses the levels of sodium, potassium, bicarbonate, and chloride.

11. **Describe the components of a basic metabolic panel.**
The basic panel includes the following components: sodium (Na^+), potassium (K^+), chloride (Cl^-), calcium (Ca^{2+}), bicarbonate (HCO_3^-), blood urea nitrogen, creatinine, and glucose.

12. **Describe the components of a comprehensive metabolic panel.**
The comprehensive metabolic panel includes the eight components that comprise the basic panel as well as albumin, total protein, alanine aminotransferase (ALT or SGPT), aspartate aminotransferase (AST or SGOT), alkaline phosphatase, and total bilirubin. At some institutions, this panel can be ordered by combining a basic metabolic panel and a set of liver function tests.

13. **What are liver function tests (LFTs)?**
Liver function tests is a term used to denote a series of assays that provide a clinician with a quick assessment of the state of liver function. Generally speaking, the components considered to be part of an LFT include AST, ALT, alkaline phosphatase, total bilirubin (fractionated into conjugated and unconjugated), albumin, and total protein.

14. **What are some commonly ordered electrolytes levels that are NOT included in the typical metabolic panels?**
Magnesium and phosphorus are the two most common additionally ordered electrolyte levels. The fluctuation in these levels is often related to the changes in other metabolite levels. Although these two electrolyte levels can often provide additional medical information, they are not used as frequently as the other components of typical metabolic panels.

15. **List the parameters assessed in a complete blood count (CBC).**
The CBC assesses red blood cell count (RBC), hemoglobin (Hgb), hematocrit (Hct), red blood indices, and white blood cell count (WBC). A CBC with a platelet count (CBCP) can also be ordered. A further component of a CBC is the differential; however, many laboratories will only perform this investigation if it is specifically requested (e.g., CBC plus diff).

16. **Specify and define the various red blood cell indices.**
Red blood cell indices are directly measured or derived values that provide information regarding the size and oxygen-carrying capacity of red blood cells. They are included as part of a routine CBC and are useful in the diagnosis of anemia. The various indices in addition to their derivations are listed in Table 4-3.

TABLE 4-3. RED BLOOD INDICES DERIVATIONS

Index	Description
Mean corpuscular volume (MCV)	The average size of red blood cells (RBCs). Calculated as follows: (hematocrit [Hct]/RBC count) × 100.
Mean corpuscular hemoglobin (MCH)	The average amount of hemoglobin per RBC. Calculated as follows: ([Hgb]/RBC count) × 100.
Mean corpuscular hemoglobin concentration (MCHC)	The average concentration of hemoglobin per RBC. Calculated as follows: ([Hgb]/Hct) × 100.
RBC distribution width (RDW)	Measures the amount of variance in size in RBC population. Calculated as follows: (SD of RBC vol/mean RBC vol) × 100.

17. Discuss the purpose of a white blood cell differential. What additional information may be obtained from this test?

A differential is an automated test that provides the relative frequency of the various types of white blood cells in a given volume of a blood sample. The cell types assayed include neutrophils, lymphocytes, monocytes, basophils, and eosinophils. Results are given as an absolute count and as percentages. Additional information is often obtained in the form of a manual count in which a differential is measured via direct microscopic examination by a pathologist. A manual count is usually only performed when abnormal results are returned by automated count.

18. Depict the shorthand format commonly used for metabolic panels and the CBC.

While on the wards, residents and students will commonly be responsible for tracking several days' worth of laboratory results for multiple patients simultaneously. One way in which medical staff deals with this task is through the use of shorthand diagrams. At first glance, these diagrams may seem difficult to interpret, but with practice they will become second nature and greatly speed the creation of medical documentation and notes for rounds. The typical notations are depicted in Fig. 4-1.

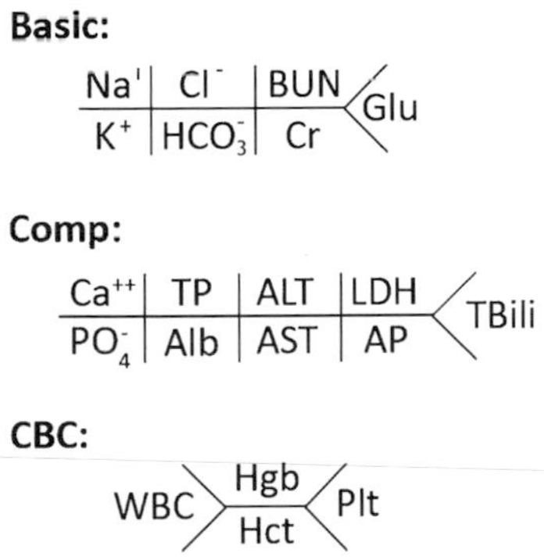

Figure 4-1. Shorthand notation for metabolic panels and complete blood cell count (CBC). *Alb*, Albumin; *ALT*, alanine aminotransferase; *AP*, alkaline phosphatase; *AST*, aspartate aminotransferase; *BUN*, blood urea nitrogen; *Ca^{++}*, calcium; *Cl^-*, chloride; *CR*, creatinine; *Glu*, glucose; *HCO_3^-*, bicarbonate; *Hct*, hematocrit; *Hgb*, hemoglobin; *K^+*, potassium; *LDH*, lactate dehydrogenase; *Na^+*, sodium; *Plt*, platelets; *PO_4^-*, phosphate; *TBili*, total bilirubin; *TP*, total protein; *WBC*, white blood cells.

19. List commonly ordered diagnostic tests by system.

A variety of commonly ordered diagnostic tests stratified by organ system are outlined in Table 4-4.

TABLE 4-4. COMMON DIAGNOSTIC TESTS BY SYSTEM

System	Diagnostic Test
Cardiovascular	Electrocardiogram (ECG), echocardiogram, stress test (dobutamine echocardiogram or nuclear medicine scan), coronary angiography (cardiac catheterization), chest x-ray (CXR), chest computed tomography (CT)/magnetic resonance imaging (MRI), 24-hour Holter monitor, event monitor, electrophysiology (EP) study, carotid doppler ultrasound, ankle-brachial indices (ABIs), orthostatic blood pressure measurement

(Continued)

TABLE 4-4. COMMON DIAGNOSTIC TESTS BY SYSTEM (CONTINUED)

System	Diagnostic Test
Pulmonary	Pulmonary function tests (PFTs)—full and spirometry, arterial blood gas (ABG), sputum gram stain and culture, bronchoscopy, bronchoalveolar lavage, tuberculin purified protein derivative (PPD) test, CXR, chest CT/MRI, pulmonary embolus (PE) protocol CT, ventilation-perfusion scan (V/Q scan)
Gastrointestinal	Barium swallow, upper endoscopy/esophagogastroduodenoscopy (EGD), upper gastrointestinal (GI) series, urea breath test, barium enema, manometry, esophageal pH monitoring, colonoscopy, sigmoidoscopy, technetium-99 m-labeled red blood cell (RBC) scintigraphy (tagged RBC scan), Hemoccult, fecal leukocytes, *Clostridium difficile* toxin, abdominal x-ray (AXR), acute abdominal series (AAS), abdominal ultrasound, abdominal CT/MRI, endoscopic retrograde cholangiopancreatography (ERCP), magnetic resonance cholangiopancreatography (MRCP), endoscopic ultrasound (EUS), percutaneous transhepatic cholangiography (PTC), hepatic 2,6-dimethyliminodiacetic acid (HIDA) scan
Renal/urologic	Kidneys-ureter-bladder x-ray (KUB), renal ultrasound, abdominal CT/MRI, intravenous pyelogram (IVP), vesicocystourethrogram (VCUG), cystoscopy, transrectal ultrasound (TRUS), renal artery ultrasound, postvoid bladder scan
Endocrinologic	Corticotropin stimulation test, dexamethasone suppression test, radioactive iodine uptake, 24-hour urine free cortisol, 24-hour aldosterone, 24-hour metanephrine/normetanephrine
Hematologic	Lower extremity Doppler ultrasound, peripheral blood smear
Obstetric/gynecologic	Glucose challenge/tolerance test, non-stress test (NST), biophysical profile (BPP), oxytocin challenge test (OCT), amniocentesis, chorionic villus sampling, percutaneous umbilical blood sampling, transabdominal ultrasound, transvaginal ultrasound, amniotic fluid index (AFI), cervical smear, whiff test
Neurologic	Electroencephalogram (EEG), electromyogram (EMG), lumbar puncture (LP), cranial x-ray, cervical spine x-ray, brain MRI/CT, brain magnetic resonance angiography (MRA)
General	Biopsy, bone scan, skeletal survey, arthrocentesis, paracentesis, thoracentesis, positron emission tomography (PET) scan

20. List the labs and diagnostic tests regularly ordered for a patient presenting with acute chest pain in the emergency department.

The typical patient presenting to the emergency department with acute-onset chest pain requires prompt evaluation to rule out several potentially life-threatening conditions. These conditions include acute coronary syndromes (i.e., unstable angina and myocardial infarction [MI]), pulmonary embolus, and aortic dissection. To effect rapid diagnosis and treatment in these situations, it is important to have an established protocol that includes laboratory and diagnostic tests in place. These laboratory tests are listed in Table 4-5 along with additional tests to consider whether clinical suspicion suggests a particular diagnosis.

TABLE 4-5. LABORATORY AND DIAGNOSTIC EVALUATION OF PATIENT WITH ACUTE CHEST PAIN

Laboratory tests	Basic metabolic panel, complete blood count (CBC), cardiac enzymes	
Diagnostic tests	Electrocardiogram (ECG), chest x-ray (CXR)	
Additional tests	Pulmonary embolus (PE)	D-dimer, lower extremity Doppler ultrasound, V/Q scan, pulmonary embolus (PE) protocol computed tomography (CT), pulmonary angiogram
	Aortic dissection	CT chest, magnetic resonance imaging (MRI), transesophageal echocardiogram (TEE)

21. **Discuss the different types of cardiac enzymes used in evaluating patients with possible myocardial ischemia.**
The term *cardiac enzymes* refers to a set of serum/plasma biomarkers (enzymes, proteins, or hormones) that are released after myocardial injury/ischemia. A rise in these biomarkers is one of two necessary components for delineating an MI (non-ST-elevation MI [NSTEMI]/ST-elevation MI [STEMI]) from myocardial ischemia (stable/unstable angina). The other necessary component is one of the following: (1) ischemic symptoms, (2) Q waves on an electrocardiogram (ECG), (3) ST elevations or depressions, or (4) coronary artery intervention such as an angioplasty.

In the emergency department (ED) or on the wards, the term cardiac enzymes generally denotes a set of laboratory tests that include troponin (trop) I or T, total creatine kinase (CK), and creatine kinase MB fraction (CK-MB). Trop is the gold standard enzyme because it has been shown to be more sensitive and specific than CK. Because CK can be released from skeletal as well as cardiac muscle, a result for the relatively cardiospecific CK-MB marker is ordered along with total CK.

Other biomarkers of cardiac injury include myoglobin, lactate dehydrogenase (LDH), AST, ALT, and heart-type fatty acid binding protein (H-FABP). However, none of these additional markers are routinely used in the diagnosis of myocardial injury.

22. **Describe the kinetics of the different cardiac enzymes.**
In the setting of myocardial injury, there is a regular rise and fall of the various cardiac enzymes. Elevations of the different enzymes occur with different lag times and the elevations persist for varying lengths of time. The kinetics of the common cardiac enzymes are characterized in Fig. 4-2.

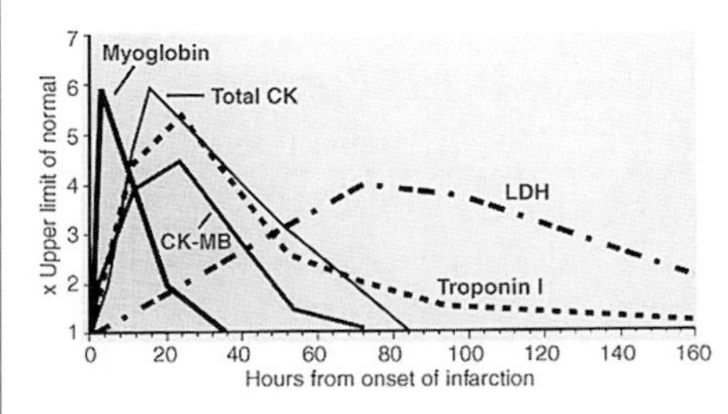

Figure 4-2. The rise and fall of cardiac enzyme levels after a myocardial infarction. (From Antman EM: General hospital management. In Julian DG, Braunwald E (eds): Management of Acute Myocardial Infarction. London, WB Saunders, 1994, with permission.)

23. What is the significance of the term *gold standard*?

The term gold standard is used to describe the single diagnostic test that is considered to be definitive for a certain disease process. In theory, this test should be 100% sensitive and 100% specific. In clinical practice there are no ideal tests, but the gold standard is thought to most closely approximate this ideal. This concept is especially important in the evaluation of new diagnostic tests via prospective/retrospective studies. In such studies, the gold standard acts as the basis for comparison of the new test and is used to generate a sensitivity/specificity. It should be noted that although it is considered the definitive test for a disease process, the gold standard is often not the most common test used. The reasons for this seeming disparity are related to issues of cost, safety, and availability. For example, consider the tests available to make a diagnosis of a pulmonary embolus. In this case, pulmonary angiography is the gold standard for diagnosis, but helical computed tomography (CT) is the most commonly used test because it is cheaper, faster, and less risky.

24. What is the utility of brain natriuretic peptide (BNP) in the management of congestive heart failure (CHF)?

BNP is a hormone released by ventricular myocardial cells in response to volume expansion and a related increase in cardiac wall stress. Logically, one would expect an increased BNP level in the volume-expanded state associated with symptomatic congestive heart failure. Therefore, BNP is frequently used to distinguish shortness of breath (SOB) due to symptomatic heart failure from pulmonary causes of SOB. It can also be used to monitor the effects of chronic treatment of heart failure as levels of BNP decrease with effective treatment. Normal values are generally <100 pg/mL, but reference ranges vary between different laboratories. BNP levels in patients with renal failure are unreliable as measures for assessing patients for CHF.

25. Outline a stepwise approach to interpreting ECGs.

- **Rate:** Divide 300 by the number of large boxes (containing 5 small boxes) between consecutive QRS complexes. 1 box = 300 bpm, 2 boxes = 150 bpm, 3 boxes = 100 bpm, 4 boxes = 75 bpm, 5 boxes = 60 bpm, etc. Normal rate is between 60 and 100 bpm.
- **Rhythm:** If every QRS complex is preceded by a P wave and every P wave is followed by a QRS complex, sinus rhythm is present. If consecutive QRS complexes are equidistant, rhythm is regular.
- **Axis:** Examine the directionality of the QRS complex in leads I and aVF. When the area above the horizontal is greater than the area below the horizontal, there is net positive QRS deflection. When the area above the horizontal is less than the area below the horizontal, there is a net negative QRS deflection. Lead I and aVF findings and the corresponding net axis determination are summarized in Table 4-6.

TABLE 4-6. ELECTROCARDIOGRAM AXIS DETERMINATION

Lead I	Lead aVF	Axis
+	+	Normal axis (+30° to −90°)
−	+	Right axis deviation
+	−	Left axis deviation
−	−	Extreme axis deviation

- **Intervals:** Important intervals to examine include the PR interval, QRS interval, and the QT interval. Measurement of these intervals, normal values, and associated pathologic conditions is outlined in Table 4-7.

TABLE 4-7. IMPORTANT ELECTROCARDIOGRAM INTERVALS

Interval	Measurement	Normal Values	Associated Pathology
PR	Start of P wave to start of Q wave	0.12–0.20 second (<5 small boxes)	>0.20: Atrioventricular (AV) block, ↑vagal tone <0.12: Wolfe-Parkinson-White syndrome
QRS	Start of Q wave to end of R/S wave	<0.10 second (<3 small boxes)	Bundle branch block, ventricular rhythm (ventricular tachycardia, ventricular flutter), hyperkalemia
QT	Start of Q wave to end of T wave	>0.45 second* for men, >0.47 second for women	Drugs (amiodarone, Ia/Ic/III antiarrhythmics, tricyclic antidepressants), hypokalemia/Mg/Ca, coronary artery disease

*Value applies to corrected QT interval (QTC).

- **Atrial chamber enlargement or ventricular wall hypertrophy:** Enlargement or hypertrophy of any of the four chambers is detectable on an ECG. Table 4-8 presents the ECG findings and etiologies associated with each.
- **Q waves:** Pathologic Q waves represent a lack of electrical activity in an area of myocardial necrosis. Isolated Q waves found in III, aVR, and V_1 can be normal. Pathologic Q waves are defined as = 0.04 second wide (1 small box) and ≥0.08 second (2 small boxes) deep or one-fourth the size of the corresponding QRS complex. These tend to be found in multiple consecutive leads corresponding to the location of the infarction (i.e., II/III/aVF = inferior, I/V_{5-6}/aVL = lateral, V_{1-2} = septal, V_{3-4} = anterior)
- **ST depressions:** This finding is usually related to subendocardial ischemia or infarction. They are generally accompanied by T wave abnormalities (e.g., T wave inversions). They also may be seen in digoxin toxicity or hypokalemia.
- **ST elevations:** This finding is related to transmural myocardial infarction. They are generally accompanied by T wave abnormalities (e.g., T wave inversions). Also, they may be seen in pericarditis, which is characterized by diffuse ST elevations in nearly every lead. Although ST elevations are generally transient, persistent ST elevations are seen when an aneurysm develops after an acute MI.
- **T wave inversions:** This finding usually represents myocardial ischemia and is generally seen in conjunction with ST elevations or depressions. Other causes of T wave inversions include chronic pericarditis/myocarditis, myocardial contusion due to trauma, and digoxin.

TABLE 4-8. ECG CHAMBER ENLARGEMENT ASSESSMENT

Chamber	ECG Findings	Etiologies
RA	V_1: Biphasic P with large (+) first portion II: P >2.5 mm in height	Suggests more serious right ventricular/ pulmonary disease
LA	V_2: Biphasic P with large (−) second portion II: P >120 msec in length	Suggests more serious left ventricular disease
RVH	V_1: R > S or R > 7 mm RAD/wide QRS	Cor pulmonale, mitral stenosis, tricuspid regurgitation, congenital L to R cardiac shunt
LVH	V_1 S + $V_{5\ or\ 6}$ R: >35 mm aVL R>11 mm LAD/wide QRS	Hypertension, aortic insufficiency, aortic stenosis, hypertrophic cardiomyopathy

LA, Left atrium; *LAD,* left anterior descending artery; *LVH,* left ventricular hypertrophy; *RA,* right atrium; *RAD,* right anterior descending artery; *RVH,* right ventricular hypertrophy.

26. What is the difference between the QT and QT_c interval?

The QT interval represents the time elapsed during a single ventricular depolarization (QRS complex) and repolarization (T wave). These events are hastened by an increased heart rate, thus decreasing the measured QT interval. Therefore, to evaluate for QT prolongation independent of the effects of heart rate, one must use the corrected QT interval (QT_c). QT_c is calculated according to the following formula: $QT_c = QT/\sqrt{R\text{-}R}$, where R-R = measured R-R interval (time between QRS complexes).

27. Compare and contrast a 24-hour Holter monitor and an event monitor.

Both devices are portable ECG monitors used for extended evaluation of rhythm abnormalities on an outpatient basis. They both record using only 2–3 leads, as opposed to the 12 leads used in an ECG. As the name implies, the 24-hour Holter monitor is used only for a 24-hour period, whereas an event monitor is used for a much longer period on the order of weeks to months (generally ≈1 month). The other main difference is related to data recording. The Holter monitor records continuously for 24 hours. In contrast, the event monitor records ECG tracings only when triggered to do so by the patient, usually when he or she is having symptoms.

Holter monitors are useful when a patient is thought to be having frequent episodes of arrhythmias or has unrecognizable/asymptomatic rhythm disturbances. In contrast, event monitors tend to be used in patients having infrequent, but symptomatic, rhythm disturbances. The goal in this case is simply to capture a single episode to help determine further diagnostic studies and proper management.

28. Review the different types of noninvasive diagnostic tests for coronary artery disease (CAD).

Noninvasive diagnostic testing for CAD is an umbrella term that encompasses many modalities for assessing the extent and effect of coronary disease. It has broad applications both in the diagnosis of new CAD and in the assessment, risk stratification, and localization of CAD in patients with documented disease. In simplified terms, in such testing "stress" is generated on the heart through the induction of increased metabolic needs. The resulting effects of this hypermetabolic state are then assessed through an ECG or imaging techniques. Table 4-9 shows the means by which the various stressors induce cardiac stress. The different methods for detecting CAD manifestations after stress are outlined in Table 4-10 and different combinations available for noninvasive CAD testing are reviewed in Table 4-11.

TABLE 4-9. STRESSORS IN NONINVASIVE CARDIAC TESTING

Stress	Mechanism
Exercise	Cardiac work is increased via ambulation on a treadmill or riding a stationary bicycle at a set speed and incline.
Dobutamine	Cardiac work is increased pharmacologically via direct stimulation of β_1-adrenergic receptors that increased heart rate and myocardial contractility.
Adenosine/ Dipyridamole (Persantine)	Cardiac stress is induced via preferential shunting of blood flow away from diseased areas. These agents are coronary vasodilators and act to increase blood flow through nondiseased coronary arteries (with normal vasodilatory capacity) and thus "steal" blood flow from diseased coronary arteries (with reduced vasodilatory capacity).

TABLE 4-10. CORONARY ARTERY DISEASE EVALUATION METHODS

Method	Positive Test Results
Physiologic parameters	Symptomatic angina, blood pressure decrease, exercise capacity <6 METS (1 MET = 3.5 mL of O_2 consumption/kg body weight/min).
ECG	Tracings indicative of ongoing myocardial ischemia. Include ST depression ≥2 mm, ST elevations, and ventricular tachycardia.
Nuclear imaging	Uptake of radioactive tracer (either thallium-201 or technetium-99 m sestamibi) by myocardial tissue. Perfusion defects (ischemia or infarction) delineated by decreased uptake.
Echocardiography	Direct visualization of cardiac motion. Ischemia or infarction evidenced by wall motion abnormality (reduced wall motion).

TABLE 4-11. MODALITIES OF NONINVASIVE CORONARY ARTERY DISEASE TESTING

Stress	Assessment Tool	Notes
Exercise	Physiologic parameters/ electrocardiogram (ECG)	Contraindicated in patients with recent myocardial infarction (<48 hours), decompensated congestive heart failure, severe arrhythmias, or severe aortic stenosis.
	Nuclear imaging	Same contraindications as above. Improved sensitivity and specificity, but also increased cost compared with exercise stress with ECG monitoring.
	Echocardiography	Same contraindication as above. Cheaper and less invasive than nuclear imaging. Lower sensitivity, but high specificity compared with nuclear imaging.

(Continued)

TABLE 4-11. MODALITIES OF NONINVASIVE CORONARY ARTERY DISEASE TESTING (CONTINUED)

Stress	Assessment Tool	Notes
Adenosine	Nuclear imaging	Used in patients unable to exercise. Demonstrates anatomic stenoses, but not active ischemia. Contraindicated in patients with hypotension, sick sinus syndrome, high-grade heart block, and severe bronchospastic disease. Make sure patients do not intake caffeine for 24 hours before test.
Dobutamine	Nuclear imaging Echocardiography	Used in patient unable to exercise. More physiologic than adenosine stress. Demonstrates presence of active stenoses. Make sure patients hold their β-blocker on the day of the stress test.

29. **What is the standard invasive method for evaluating CAD?**

Coronary angiography is currently the gold standard for invasive evaluation of CAD. The procedure involves the injection of a radiopaque dye via a catheter fed from a peripheral artery (usually the femoral artery) into the coronary ostia. Fluoroscopy (real-time x-ray) is then used to visualize the flow of the dye through the coronary arteries. Diseased vessels are detected as narrowings of dye flow through a vessel. This procedure does have significant associated risks including stroke, MI, bleeding, infection, and arterial dissection. Newer, although unproven, methods of noninvasive coronary angiography are currently available, but are in limited use. They include CT and magnetic resonance coronary angiography.

30. **List the laboratory and diagnostic tests regularly ordered for a patient presenting with acute dyspnea in the ED.**

The patient presenting to the ED with acute dyspnea may be suffering from a pulmonary or cardiac condition, conditions leading to acid/base disturbances, or other less likely conditions. Pulmonary causes of acute dyspnea to consider include pulmonary embolus (PE), acute pneumonia, pneumothorax, asthma, chronic obstructive pulmonary disease (COPD) exacerbation, or aspiration/ acute respiratory distress syndrome (ARDS). Cardiac causes include MI, CHF exacerbation, pericardial tamponade, or an acute arrhythmia. Other possible causes include carbon monoxide poisoning, acute anemia, sepsis, or panic attack. To promptly evaluate such patients, it is best to have a protocol including laboratory and diagnostic tests in mind. Table 4-12 shows a list of such a set of laboratory/diagnostic tests and includes additional tests to consider on the basis of increased clinical suspicion (according to history/physical examination) for a particular condition.

TABLE 4-12. LABORATORY AND DIAGNOSTIC EVALUATIONS TO CONSIDER IN A PATIENT WITH ACUTE DYSPNEA

Laboratory tests	Basic metabolic panel, complete blood count (CBC), cardiac enzymes, brain natriuretic peptide (BNP)	
Diagnostic tests	Arterial blood gas (ABG), chest x-ray (CXR), electrocardiogram (ECG), computed tomography (CT), echocardiogram (ECHO)	
Additional tests	Pulmonary embolus (PE)	D-dimer, lower extremity Doppler ultrasound, V/Q scan, PE protocol CT
	Sepsis	Blood culture

31. Discuss the indications for arterial blood gas (ABG) analysis.

With the advent of pulse oximetry for the determination of arterial hemoglobin saturation, the indications for arterial blood gas analysis have become blurred. Nonetheless, several clinical scenarios demand the use of this diagnostic test including (1) the firm determination of the severity of oxygenation deficit, (2) the evaluation of hypo- or hyperventilation (e.g., P_aCO_2), (3) the evaluation of acid-base status, and (4) the maintenance of patients receiving chronic mechanical ventilation.

32. List the elements assayed in an ABG analysis.

Directly measured:

- pH = measure of acidemia or alkalinemia
- P_aO_2 = partial pressure of oxygen in arterial blood
- P_aCO_2 = partial pressure of carbon dioxide in arterial blood

Calculated:

- O_2 sat = percentage of hemoglobin saturated with oxygen in arterial blood
- HCO_3^- = concentration of bicarbonate in blood
- Base excess/deficit = sum total of metabolic buffering agents (anions such as HCO_3^-) in blood

33. Describe the key concepts in the interpretation of an ABG analysis regarding oxygenation and ventilation.

To interpret ABG values, one must first understand the two key features of pulmonary function: oxygenation and ventilation. Oxygenation refers to the maintenance of an adequate oxygen partial pressure such that hemoglobin is appropriately saturated. Ventilation refers to the act of replacing old, noxious air with fresh, oxygenated air. The five mechanisms leading to inadequate oxygenation are listed in Table 4-13 along with common pathologic conditions that act by the corresponding mechanism. ABG analysis is essential in determining which mechanism is responsible for inadequate oxygenation and thus can suggest an underlying pathologic condition. The relationship between the elements assayed in an ABG analysis and mechanisms of hypoxia are listed in Table 4-14.

TABLE 4-13. MECHANISMS OF INADEQUATE OXYGENATION

Mechanism	Associated Pathology
Low inspired O_2	High altitude
Hypoventilation	↓ respiratory drive (i.e. neurologic), neuropathies (i.e., amyotrophic lateral sclerosis), neuromuscular junction disease (i.e., myasthenia gravis), myopathy (i.e., muscular dystrophies), chest wall abnormalities
Diffusion impairment	Interstitial lung disease, pulmonary edema, acute respiratory distress syndrome
V/Q mismatch	Asthma, chronic obstructive pulmonary disease, pneumonia, congestive heart failure, pulmonary embolus
True shunt	Intrapulmonary shunt (i.e., arteriovenous malformation), right-to-left cardiac shunt

TABLE 4-14. ARTERIAL BLOOD GAS INTERPRETATIONS

Mechanism	P_aO_2	P_aCO_2	A-a gradient	Response to 100% O_2
Low inspired O_2	↓	↓	Normal	↑ P_aO_2
Hypoventilation	↓	↑	Normal	↓ P_aO_2
Diffusion impairment	↓	Normal	↑	↑ P_aO_2
V/Q mismatch	↓	Normal	↑	↑ P_aO_2
True shunt	↓	Normal	↑	No change

A-a gradient, Alveolar-arterial gradient; *$PaCO_2$,* partial pressure of carbon dioxide in arterial blood; *PaO_2,* partial pressure of oxygen in arterial blood.

An important concept used here is the alveolar-arterial gradient, also known as the *A-a gradient*. It is calculated using the measured components of an ABG analysis according to the following formula $([P_AO_2] - [P_aO_2]) = [F_iO_2 \times (760 - 47) - (P_aCO_2/0.8)] - [P_aO_2]$. The normal A-a gradient = (age/4) + 4. An additional important concept of which to be aware is the relationship between P_aCO_2 and ventilation. Acutely, CO_2 can only be eliminated via expiration; thus the P_aCO_2 is inversely proportional to the degree ventilation (i.e., ↑ P_aCO_2 = ↓ ventilation).

34. Outline a general stepwise approach to interpreting acid-base status from an ABG.

- **Acidemic versus Alkalotic**
  pH <7.35 = acidemic
  pH >7.45 = alkalemic
- **Respiratory versus Metabolic**
  Acidemic + P_aCO_2 >40 = respiratory acidosis
  Acidemic + HCO_3^- <22 = metabolic acidosis
  Alkalemic + HCO_3^- >26 = metabolic alkalosis
  Alkalemic + P_aCO_2 <40 = respiratory alkalosis
- **Acute versus Chronic** (respiratory acidosis/alkalosis only) (only a general rule of thumb)
  Acute acidosis/alkalosis: $\Delta pH = 0.08 \times [(P_aCO_2 - 40)/10]$
  Chronic acidosis/alkalosis: $\Delta pH = 0.03 \times [(P_aCO_2 - 40)/10]$
  Note: decreased effect of ↑ or ↓ P_aCO_2 in chronic acidosis/alkalosis due to increased production of HCO_3^- in acidosis and increased renal elimination of HCO_3^- in alkalosis. This process takes time, however, and thus is seen only in chronic acid-base disturbances.
- **Adequacy of compensation**
  - **Respiratory acidosis**
  Acute: ↑ $HCO_3^- = \Delta P_aCO_2/10$
  Chronic: ↑ $HCO_3^- = 4 \times \Delta P_aCO_2/10$
  - **Respiratory alkalosis**
  Acute: ↑ $HCO_3^- = 2 \times \Delta P_aCO_2/10$
  Chronic: ↑ $HCO_3^- = 4 \times \Delta P_aCO_2/10$
  Note: if inadequate compensation or overcompensation is present, a mixed acid-base disorder is present (i.e., more than a single disturbance such as metabolic acidosis and respiratory alkalosis).

- **Anion gap**
  Anion gap (AG) = $Na^+ - (Cl^- + HCO_3^-)$
  Note: normal values = 8-12 mEq/L; values exceeding 14 = anion gap metabolic acidosis
- **Change in bicarbonate versus anion gap** (anion gap metabolic acidosis only)
  If AG >20, then a metabolic acidosis is present regardless of pH or HCO_3^-.
  If AG is high, then calculate the excess AG (AG-12).
  Add this to the HCO_3^- that was measured, and:
  If the sum is >30, then there is an underlying metabolic alkalosis is present.
  If the sum is <23, then an underlying non-anion gap metabolic acidosis is present.

35. **Outline a stepwise approach to interpreting chest x-rays.**
When examining a chest x-ray on the wards, the temptation is to immediately stare at one or both lung fields in the hopes of spotting an obvious pulmonary finding. This technique will often lead to multiple errors in interpretation including missing key findings. Also, a stepwise approach demonstrates to senior residents and staff that the film is being examined thoroughly. The following stepwise approach will assure that all areas of the film are covered. *Note:* for help remembering the various steps in this examination, think of the mnemonic, "**A**re **T**here **M**any **L**ung **L**esions?"
- ***A*bdomen:** Examine the areas below the diaphragm. Assess whether diaphragms are flattened (COPD/asthma) or asymmetric. Elevated hemidiaphragms indicate ipsilateral atelectasis, diaphragmatic paralysis, or a subdiaphragmatic process (abdominal abscess or hematoma). Be especially alert for pneumoperitoneum (air under the diaphragm) indicating perforated bowel.
- ***T*horax:** Examine the bones and soft tissues that constitute the thorax. These include the ribs and axillary/shoulder soft tissue. Be alert for subcutaneous emphysema and rib fractures.
- ***M*ediastinum:** Examine the pharynx, trachea, carina, and cardiac silhouette. Be alert for shifts in tracheal position (tension pneumothorax), upper airway foreign bodies (metallic), widened mediastinum (aortic dissection), and enlarged hearts (CHF or tamponade).
- ***L*ungs alone:** Examine the lungs individually. Be alert for air-fluid levels (pneumonia), pleural effusions, interstitial/alveolar edema (CHF or ARDS), hyperinflation (COPD), and solitary pulmonary nodules (lung cancer or tuberculosis).
- ***L*ungs together:** Examine the lungs together. Be alert for the same entities as in the preceding point.

36. **Describe the alternative ABCDEFGH approach to interpreting chest x-rays.**
- ***A*ssessment/*A*irway:** Evaluate the quality of the film. Is there adequate inspiration? Counting eight or more ribs assures good inspiration. Is the film under- or overexposed? Assess the detail of the spine to determine exposure. Excessive spinal detail (spine is very white) indicates overexposure. No spinal detail (spine is not visible) indicates underexposure. Is the patient rotated? Assess rotation by evaluating the positions of the clavicles. Assess the airway by looking for whether the trachea is midline or shifted to one side.
- ***B*ones/Soft Tissue:** Scan for rib fractures, decreased bone density, or bony metastatic lesions. Look in subcutaneous tissue for air or foreign bodies.
- ***C*ardiac:** Examine cardiac silhouette for enlargement and the presence of calcifications. Note any irregularities in shape (globular = pericarditis/tamponade).
- ***D*iaphragm:** Examine diaphragms for flattening or asymmetry. Be wary of air underneath the diaphragm.

- ***E*ffusions:** Pleural effusions are most recognizable via the opacification of a hemithorax and blunting of lateral costophrenic angles.
- ***F*ields:** Evaluate bilateral lung fields for the presence of infiltrates/consolidation (pneumonia, CHF, ARDS, or hemorrhage) and absent (pneumothorax) or increased vascular markings (CHF).
- ***G*reat Vessels:** Assess for increased aortic size (aortic dissection) or aortic calcifications (CAD). Evaluate for increase pulmonary artery size (CHF, pulmonary hypertension).
- ***H*ila/Mediastinum:** Scan for hilar lymphadenopathy (sarcoidosis) or calcifications (sarcoidosis), as well as for any mediastinal widening (aortic dissection).

37. What is the upper limit of normal for the cardiac silhouette on chest x-rays?

Generally speaking, cardiac silhouettes exceeding 50% of the thoracic diameter on an anteroposterior (AP) film are considered enlarged. Alternatively, an increase in the diameter of the cardiac silhouette by >1 cm defines an acute cardiac enlargement. Of course, both of these descriptions are subject to debate, and there is some controversy among radiologists about the sensitivity/specificity of this designation. However, to be safe assume that the heart should not take up more space than half the width of the thorax. It is important to be sure to assess an AP film rather than a posteroanterior (PA) film because the heart appears larger on a PA film.

38. List the laboratory and diagnostic tests regularly ordered for a patient presenting with acute abdominal pain in the ED.

The patient presenting to the emergency department with acute abdominal pain may have any of myriad collection of disorders affecting the gastrointestinal (GI), genitourinary, and musculoskeletal systems. Although appendicitis remains the most frequent cause of an acute abdomen in the United States, other common etiologies—cholecystitis, hepatitis, pancreatitis, pyelonephritis, nephrolithiasis, diverticulitis, ectopic pregnancies, and pelvic inflammatory disease—must be considered when initial laboratory and diagnostic tests are ordered. Because of the diverse set of etiologies responsible for the acute abdomen, the history and physical examination plays a much more prominent role in guiding the selection of appropriate tests than in more focused complaints such as chest pain or acute dyspnea. A set of commonly ordered laboratory and diagnostic tests used in evaluating patients presenting with acute abdominal pain is shown in Table 4-15.

TABLE 4-15. LABORATORY AND DIAGNOSTIC EVALUATION OF PATIENT WITH ACUTE ABDOMINAL PAIN

Laboratory tests	Comprehensive metabolic panel, complete blood count (CBC), amylase/lipase, urinalysis, pregnancy test
Diagnostic tests	Acute abdominal series, abdominal and pelvic computed tomography (CT) scan
Additional tests	Cholecystitis, diverticulitis, right upper quadrant ultrasound, abdominal CT

39. Describe the components and purpose of an acute abdominal x-ray series (AAS).

An AAS, also called the *three-way abdomen,* consists of upright chest, upright abdominal, and supine abdominal radiographs. It is commonly used in the diagnosis of bowel obstructions and adynamic ileus, which are characterized by the presence of distended, gas-filled bowel loops, and multiple air-fluid levels. As this name implies, this radiographic series has some diagnostic use in patients presenting with acute abdominal pain; however, with the advent of cheap, fast, and readily available CT technology, unenhanced helical CT has largely replaced the AAS because of its superior sensitivity.

40. Describe the similarities and differences between a barium swallow, an upper GI series, and a small bowel series.

Each of these studies involves the oral ingestion of barium contrast material. The progress of the contrast material is tracked by a series of plain radiographs or fluoroscopic images. The studies differ in the areas assessed by radiography. The barium swallow is used to evaluate the esophagus alone, whereas an upper GI series images the esophagus, stomach, and duodenum. A small bowel series evaluates the small bowel from the duodenojejunal junction to the ileocecal valve. Each of these studies can be used to detect a wide variety of pathologic conditions in their respective distributions. Important diagnostic findings include ulcers, polyps, tumors, obstructions, strictures, and inflammatory bowel disease.

41. Discuss the significance of the various components included in the liver function tests (LFTs).

LFTs are used largely for the detection and differentiation of three types of liver pathologic conditions: (1) hepatocellular injury, (2) cholestasis, and (3) decreased synthetic function. To get a more robust evaluation for these pathologic conditions, traditional LFTs (AST, ALT, alkaline phosphatase, total protein, albumin, and total bilirubin) are supplemented with additional tests including coagulation test (PT/international normalized ratio (INR)), glucose, and γ-glutamyltransferase. The expected derangements in these laboratory tests with each of the three aforementioned pathologic conditions are outlined in Table 4-16. Related disease processes are also included.

TABLE 4-16. LABORATORY ABNORMALITIES ASSOCIATED WITH LIVER DISEASE

Liver Pathology	Laboratory Tests	Related Disease Processes
Hepatocellular injury	↑ AST/↑ ALT ± ↑ AP ↑ Tbili	Viral hepatitis, autoimmune hepatitis, toxic hepatitis, alcoholic liver disease, neoplasm
Cholestasis	↑ AP/↑ GGT ± ↑ AST/↑ ALT ↑ Tbili	Biliary obstruction (choledocholithiasis, cholecystitis, etc.), infiltrative disease (neoplastic, granulomatous)
↓ Synthetic function	↑ PT ↓ Albumin ↓ Glucose ↓ BUN	Any of the above disease processes; generally hepatocellular injury leads to greater decrements in synthetic function compared with cholestatic disease

ALT, Alanine aminotransferase; *AP,* alkaline phosphatase; *AST,* aspartate alanine aminotransferase; *BUN,* blood urea nitrogen; *GGT,* γ-glutamyltransferase; *PT,* total protein; *Tbili,* total bilirubin.

42. List the laboratory and diagnostic tests regularly ordered for patient presenting with acute renal failure.

In addition to supportive measures, the key to managing acute renal failure lies in the treatment of the underlying cause. Thus, the elucidation of the type of renal failure—prerenal, intrinsic renal, or postrenal—is an important step in the determination of a precise etiology. Along with a thorough history and physical examination focused on comorbid diseases and current medications, a standard set of laboratory and diagnostic tests is essential in helping to determine the type of renal failure. A set of commonly ordered laboratory and diagnostic tests used in evaluating patients presenting with acute renal failure is shown in Table 4-17.

TABLE 4-17. LABORATORY AND DIAGNOSTIC EVALUATION OF PATIENT WITH ACUTE RENAL FAILURE

Laboratory tests	Basic metabolic panel, complete blood count (CBC), urinalysis, urine electrolytes (Na^+, K^+, Cl^-), urine osmolarity, urine creatinine
Diagnostic tests	Renal ultrasound, postvoid residual

43. Discuss the interpretation of urine electrolytes, osmolarity, and creatinine in regard to acute renal failure.

Measurements of urine electrolytes, osmolarity, and creatinine are commonly used in differentiating prerenal from renal causes of acute renal failure. An important concept in this determination is that of the fractional excretion of sodium (FeNa). The FeNa is a measure of the percentage of sodium excreted in the urine compared with the total amount of urine entering the renal tubules. It is calculated according to the following equation ($Urine_{Na} \times Plasma_{Cr}$)/($Plasma_{Na} \times Urine_{Cr}$). A list of the values of FeNa along with those of several other urine electrolyte-based measures that suggest prerenal versus intrinsic renal failure is shown in Table 4-18.

TABLE 4-18. URINE ELECTROLYTE VALUES IN ACUTE PRERENAL VERSUS INTRINSIC RENAL FAILURE

Measure	Prerenal	Renal
FeNa (%)	<1	>3
Urine osmolarity	>500	<350
Urine sodium	<20	>40
Urine Cr/Plasma Cr	>40	<20

Cr, Creatinine; *FeNa,* fractional excretion of sodium.

To understand the physiology driving these differences, one should consider a patient with acute prerenal failure due to hypovolemia and compare him or her to a patient with acute intrinsic renal failure due to acute tubular necrosis. In the hypovolemic patient, the renal tubular epithelial cells continue to function and thus are actively reabsorbing sodium to conserve as much volume (H_2O) as possible. Thus, the fractional sodium excretion is low, the total urinary sodium is low, and, because of the intense efforts by the tubular cells to reabsorb maximal H_2O, the urine osmolarity is high (i.e., the urine is concentrated). The opposite is true in the case of acute tubular necrosis because of the dysfunction of renal tubular epithelial cells, which are necrotic or ischemic.

44. What is the fractional excretion of urea?

Diuretics affect the excretion of sodium. In patients receiving diuretics, FeNa may therefore not be the best parameter for determining the cause of acute renal failure. Transport of urea is not affected by diuretics, so in these patients a fractional excretion of urea (Fe_{urea}), calculated as ($Urine_{urea} \times Plasma_{Cr}$)/($Plasma_{urea} \times Urine_{Cr}$), <35% is suggestive of a prerenal etiology of acute renal failure.

45. Discuss the interpretation of urinary pH in regards to renal tubular acidosis.

Renal tubular acidosis (RTA) is a set of medical conditions characterized by non–anion gap acidosis due to failure of the kidneys to properly acidify the urine. One should consider RTA in the differential diagnosis of a patient who presents with non–anion gap acidosis and does not have GI symptoms. There are three different mechanisms whereby the kidneys fail to properly acidify the urine, which have been designated type I RTA, type II RTA, and type IV RTA. As the treatments for the different types of RTA differ slightly, it is necessary to delineate the type of RTA present in a patient. Furthermore, the underlying causes of the renal defects differ among the different RTAs; thus, ascertaining the type of RTA can help pin down a cause of the defect. Interpreting urinary pH and serum electrolytes is the key step in delineating the type of RTA. The values of urinary pH and urinary K that are associated with the different RTAs and suggested etiologies to consider are outlined in Table 4-19.

TABLE 4-19. URINARY pH AND ELECTROLYTES IN RENAL TUBULAR ACIDOSIS

Type	Urine pH	Serum K	Etiologies
I	>5.3	Low	[Failure to secrete H^+ in distal tubules] Hereditary, autoimmune (Sjögren, systemic lupus erythematosus, rheumatoid arthritis), medication (amphotericin B, lithium), cirrhosis
II	<5.3	Low	[Failure to resorb HCO_3^- in proximal tubules] Hereditary (Fanconi syndrome, Wilson disease, cystinosis), heavy metal poisoning, multiple myeloma, amyloidosis, medications (highly active antiretroviral treatment, ifosfamide, carbonic anhydrase inhibitors)
IV	<5.3	High	[Hyporeninemic hypoaldosteronism] Chronic kidney disease due to diabetes mellitus/hypertension/human immunodeficiency virus infection/medications, chronic urinary tract obstruction, mediations (angiotensin-converting enzyme inhibitors, potassium-sparing diuretics)

46. Discuss the significance of the various components of a urinalysis.

A urinalysis is ordered to evaluate for a vast array of disorders, including urinary tract infections, kidney stones, renal failure, nephrotic syndrome, diabetic ketoacidosis, and biliary disease. The components commonly included in a urinalysis and associated possible interpretations are listed in Table 4-20.

TABLE 4-20. INTERPRETING A URINALYSIS

Component	Findings	Interpretation
Appearance	Clear	Normal
	Cloudy	Pyuria, lipiduria, hyperoxaluria
Color	Clear to yellow	Normal
	Red/tea-colored	Hematuria, hemoglobinuria, myoglobinuria
	Brown/black	Bile pigments
	Orange	Rifampin use, pyridium use
Urine pH	Alkaline	Urinary tract infection (UTI) due to urease-positive bacteria, struvite calculi
	Acidic	Uric acid calculi
Specific gravity	Elevated	Dehydration, syndrome of inappropriate antidiuretic hormone (SIADH), glycosuria
	Decreased	Diuretic use, diabetes insipidus, adrenal insufficiency, hypoaldosteronism, impaired renal function
Blood	Positive	Nephrolithiasis, cystitis/pyelonephritis, urologic neoplasm, urologic trauma, nephritis (e.g., IgA nephropathy, rapidly progressive glomerulonephritis)
Protein	Elevated	Exercise, fever, diabetes mellitus, congestive heart failure, multiple myeloma, amyloidosis, nephrotic/nephritic syndrome
Leukocyte esterase	Positive	UTI (Note: produced by responding neutrophils)
Nitrite	Positive	UTI (Note: produced by bacterial reduction of nitrates to nitrites; however, not all bacteria are capable of this reduction, just the common ones such as *Escherichia coli*)
Glucose	Positive	Diabetes mellitus, Cushing syndrome, Fanconi syndrome
Ketones	Positive	Diabetic ketoacidosis, uncontrolled diabetes mellitus, starvation
Bilirubin	Elevated	Hepatocellular disease, biliary obstruction
Urobilinogen	Elevated	Hemolysis, hepatocellular disease
	Decreased	Biliary obstruction

47. List the common 24-hour urine collection assays and the conditions for which they are used as diagnostic tools.

The various assays for which 24-hour urine samples are collected and analyzed in addition to detailing common conditions for which these tests have diagnostic implications are reviewed in Table 4-21.

TABLE 4-21. 24-HOUR URINE COLLECTION ASSAYS

Factor Assayed	Diagnostic Implications
Electrolytes (sodium, potassium, chloride, calcium, magnesium, phosphorus)	Acute/chronic renal failure
Creatinine/blood urea nitrogen	Acute/chronic renal failure
Glucose	Diabetes mellitus
Protein	Nephrotic syndrome, multiple myeloma, Waldenström hypergammaglobulinemia, diabetes mellitus, lupus, amyloidosis, pre-eclampsia
Free cortisol	Cushing syndrome
Aldosterone	Primary hyperaldosteronism (Conn syndrome)
Metanephrine/normetanephrine	Pheochromocytoma
Uric acid/oxalate/cysteine	Renal calculi predisposition
Hydroxyproline	Increased bone resorption (Paget disease, osteoporosis, multiple myeloma, hyperthyroidism)
Copper/lead/mercury/arsenic/cadmium	Heavy metal toxicity

48. List the laboratory and diagnostic tests commonly used to evaluate suspected thyroid disease.

Thyroid dysfunction is a commonly encountered problem in the outpatient setting. Hypo- or hyperthyroidism can oftentimes be diagnosed solely on the basis of historical and physical findings; however, determining the underlying cause usually requires a comprehensive set of laboratory and diagnostic tests. The components of a typical set of tests to evaluate thyroid dysfunction are listed in Table 4-22.

TABLE 4-22. LABORATORY AND DIAGNOSTIC EVALUATION OF PATIENT WITH SUSPECTED THYROID DYSFUNCTION

Laboratory tests	Thyroid function tests (TSH, free T_3/T_4), comprehensive metabolic panel, complete blood count (CBC), antithyroid antibodies (anti-TPO), creatine kinase, lipid panel. Note: TSH is the initial screening test.	
Diagnostic tests	Thyroid ultrasound, thyroid uptake/scintigraphy, T_3 resin uptake	
Additional tests	Thyroid nodule	Fine-needle aspiration
	Graves disease	Thyroid-stimulating antibodies

TSH, Thyroid-stimulating hormone, *T_3*, triiodothyronine, *T_4*, thyroxine.

49. Discuss the use of radionuclide testing in the diagnosis of thyroid disease.
Radionuclide testing plays an important role in diagnosing thyroid disease and is used in two major tests of thyroid function: (1) thyroid uptake/scintigraphy and (2) triiodothyronine (T_3) resin uptake. Thyroid scintigraphy is based on the fact that iodine serves as the precursor for the production of thyroid hormone. As the thyroid becomes more or less active in the production of thyroid hormone (i.e., in hyper- and hypothyroid states), more iodine is taken up into the thyroid gland and used in the production of this hormone. Scintigraphy works by injecting radiolabeled iodine (iodine-123) or technetium-99 m and imaging the distribution of the radiolabel in the thyroid This test is especially useful in delineating diffuse (e.g., Graves) from multifocal (e.g., multinodular goiter) thyroid disease, which can be difficult to do clinically. Table 4-23 lists the physical examination and thyroid scintigraphy findings associated with commonly encountered thyroid conditions.

TABLE 4-23. THYROID DISEASE AND ASSOCIATED CLINICAL AND DIAGNOSTIC FINDINGS

Thyroid Condition	Clinical Findings	Radioiodine Scan
Graves disease	Diffusely enlarged; painless	↑ diffuse uptake (homogenous)
Multinodular toxic goiter	Multiple nodules; painless	↑ diffuse uptake (heterogeneous)
Toxic adenoma	Single nodule; painless	↑ focal uptake
Hashimoto thyroiditis	Diffusely enlarged; painless	↓ uptake
Subacute thyroiditis	Diffusely enlarged; painful	↓ uptake

T_3 resin uptake is a second test of thyroid function that employs radionuclides. As opposed to the thyroid uptake scan, this test is done in vitro. In this test, radiolabeled T_3 is added to a sample of the patient's serum. After a period of incubation, resin is added. The amount of radiolabeled T_3 bound to the resin is subsequently measured, giving an indirect measure of the amount of thyroid-binding globulin (TBG) present in a patent's serum. The greater the amount of radiolabeled T_3 bound to the resin, the lower the level of endogenous TBG in the patient's serum. The test works because as the amount of TBG in a sample increases, there are more sites for the radiolabeled T_3 to bind to. Thus, when the resin is added, there is less free T3 to bind the resin, decreasing the amount of T3 resin uptake. The TBG level is important as altered levels confound the measurement of thyroid hormone (T_3 or thyroxine). When TBG is high, the measured amount of thyroid hormone in the serum is high, even though the free (i.e., physiologically active) level of thyroid hormone is normal. This occurs because the assay for measuring thyroid hormone takes into account ALL thyroid hormone, not just the free fraction.

50. Discuss the laboratory and diagnostic evaluation of a patient presenting with abnormal bleeding.
The initial evaluation of a patient with abnormal bleeding involves a large set of tests; however, narrowing the differential diagnosis can be accomplished by concentrating on three parameters: (1) PT, (2) aPTT, and (3) bleeding time. Abnormal PT and aPTT indicate disorders related to coagulation factors, whereas an abnormal bleeding time denotes a disorder of platelets, either quantitative or qualitative. Table 4-24 outlines the permutations of disturbances in these three parameters and suggests possible associated etiologies for the abnormal bleeding on the basis of the testing results.

TABLE 4-24. PROTHROMBIN TIME (PT), ACTIVATED PARTIAL THROMBOPLASTIN TIME (aPTT), AND BLEEDING TIME IN THE EVALUATION OF ABNORMAL BLEEDING

PT	aPTT	Bleeding Time	Etiologies
↑	Normal	Normal	Liver disease, vitamin K deficiency, factor VII deficiency, early disseminated intravascular coagulation (DIC), warfarin use
Normal	↑	Normal	Hemophilia A/B, factor deficiency or presence of an inhibitor (all factors, except for factor VII), antiphospholipid antibody syndrome (presence of lupus anticoagulant), heparin use
↑	↑	Normal	DIC, severe liver disease, warfarin overdose, severe vitamin K deficiency, coagulation factor washout (massive transfusion; plasmapheresis without fresh frozen plasma)
Normal	Normal	↑	Decreased platelet count: thrombocytopenia Normal platelet count: uremia, acetylsalicylic acid/nonsteroidal anti-inflammatory drugs, myeloproliferative disease, multiple myeloma/Waldenström macroglobulinemia, antiplatelet antibody, von Willebrand disease, Bernard-Soulier syndrome, Glanzmann thrombasthenia

KEY POINTS: LABS AND DIAGNOSTIC TESTS

1. Most orders are written as routine and generally take several hours. Orders can be written as STAT to expedite the return of results.
2. Metabolic panels are commonly ordered laboratory tests that can provide informative data on the basis of electrolyte levels.
3. Many common patient presentations, such as chest pain, have associated protocols for laboratory and diagnostics tests that are specific to each institution.
4. An arterial blood gas analysis can be used to determine oxygenation deficit, evaluation of hypo- or hyperventilation, evaluation of acid-base status, and the maintenance of patients receiving chronic mechanical ventilation.
5. Two mnemonics for reading chest x-rays are "Are There Many Lung Lesions?" and the ABCDEFGH method.
6. Numerous types of laboratory and diagnostic tests are available. Each, when ordered appropriately, can provide significant information on patient status and affect future patient management.

CHAPTER 5

MEDICAL DOCUMENTATION AND WRITING ORDERS

Javier A. Valle, Mitesh S. Patel, and Joseph D. Maratt

1. **What is the purpose of the medical record?**
   The medical record is intended to provide a detailed account of the care that a patient receives and is essential for quality and continuity of care. It is also important from a billing and legal standpoint.

2. **How does documentation become part of the official medical record?**
   There are several methods for documentation in different medical centers. In many centers documentation is recorded electronically and becomes part of the official medical record as soon as it is digitally signed by the attending physician caring for the patient. In many institutions, documentation is available online before attending review if a resident physician has verified its accuracy.

3. **Who may contribute to the medical record?**
   Hospital staff involved in patient care are permitted and expected to contribute to the medical record. In some institutions, medical students are also permitted to contribute to the record. However, medical student documentation must be reviewed, edited for accuracy, and signed by a supervising staff member.

4. **What should be included in the medical record?**
   Any medical decision making, as well as the basis for those decisions, should become part of the medical record. In addition, any procedures or significant interactions should also become part of the record. In the highly litigious medical system, if you do not document it, you did not do it.

5. **What should be documented when a patient is admitted to the hospital?**
   A patient being admitted to the hospital needs a thorough admission history and physical examination. This history details the reason for the patient's admission. The accuracy of the physical examination is particularly important as it provides the baseline to which future examinations are compared. During every admission, the past medical history, past surgical history, current medications, drug allergies, family history, social history, and code status should also be reviewed and documented.

6. **What should be documented daily?**
   Daily documentation of the patient's status and care provided is essential. The elements involved are a brief history from the patient regarding changes from the previous day, a physical examination, and medical decision making. The usual format for this is a SOAP (Subjective, Objective, Assessment, and Plan) note. The components of a SOAP note are displayed in Table 5-1.

TABLE 5-1. COMPONENTS OF A SOAP NOTE

Subjective	Changes over the past day and events.
Objective	Physical examination, laboratory results, study results
Assessment	Reassessment of patient's diagnosis, treatment and condition
Plan	Updated plan for care, divided by problem or by organ system

7. **Provide an example of a daily progress note.**
Examples of typical SOAP notes for both a surgical and a medicine service are displayed in Table 5-2. Note that although both are brief, medicine notes tend to be more detailed. The "problem list" will tend to be longer and will include more chronic issues. Surgical notes tend to have shorter problem lists and will focus specifically on the surgical issue at hand. Also, surgical notes will focus on the surgical wound after a procedure. In both types of notes, any new results of diagnostic tests (e.g. laboratory tests and imaging) or therapeutic procedures should be recorded.

TABLE 5-2. THE DAILY PROGRESS NOTE

General Surgery Note Date	Medicine Progress Note Date
S: Mr. Smith's pain is well controlled with no events overnight.	**S:** Mr. Smith is doing well today, continued cough productive of yellow sputum overnight. He slept well and had no events overnight.
O: Gen: Awake, alert, NAD. CV: RRR, +S1,S2, no M/R/G. Resp: Soft crackles on the right. Abd: Soft, nondistended. No bowel sounds heard. Mild diffuse tenderness to palpation. Incisions clean, dry, and intact with staples in place. Ext: Distal pulses intact. No cyanosis or edema. CXR: Clear with no signs of pneumothorax. ECG: NSR.	**O:** Gen: Awake, alert, NAD. CV: RRR, +S1,S2, no M/R/G. Resp: crackles at right lower base, tactile fremitus to palpation on right side. Abd: Soft, nontender, nondistended. +BS. Ext: 2+ distal pulses in all 4 extremities. No cyanosis or edema. CXR: Clear with no signs of pneumothorax. ECG: NSR.
A/P: Mr. Smith is POD #1 s/p open appendectomy in stable condition. —Continue PCA —Advance diet to clears —Monitor bowel function	**A/P:** Mr. Smith is a 59 y.o. male with likely COPD exacerbation vs. PNA. 1. COPD v. PNA —Continue abx, Levaquin (day 5 of 10) —Continue O2 by NC 2. HTN —Continue home Lisinopril, HCTZ

BS, Bowel sounds; *COPD*, chronic obstructive pulmonary disorder; *CV*, cardiovascular; *CXR*, chest x-ray; *ECG*, electrocardiogram; *HCTZ*, hydrochlorothiazide; *HTN*, hypertension; *M/R/G*, murmurs, rubs, or gallops; *NAD*, no apparent distress; *NSR*, normal sinus rhythm; *PCA*, patient-controlled analgesia; *PNA*, pneumonia; *POD*, postoperative day; *RRR*, regular rate and rhythm.

8. What is an order?

An order is a single specific instruction to be implemented according to a patient's medical care protocol. Some orders may be executed only once, whereas others may be scheduled to occur at regular intervals. Examples of an order include placement of intravenous line access, addition of a medication, a blood draw, and specification of a diet.

9. How are orders managed?

Patient care orders are usually managed through a permanent record that is translated into a patient care routine. This is done in some institutions through a paper system and in others through computerized systems. Paper systems usually require one clear instruction per order line. In computerized systems, orders are usually entered through a series of prompts of possible choices. It is also possible to write "free text" orders in these systems when the prompts do not include the exact order instructions.

10. How can an order be stopped or discontinued?

In a paper system, discontinuation of an order is accomplished by stating the discontinuation of a specific instruction already in the nursing routine. For example, to stop a patient's penicillin course, you may write "D/C penicillin." In a computerized system, an order is usually discontinued by locating it in the list of standing orders and choosing the discontinue option. In some systems, you will be prompted for a reason for discontinuation. Often, the reason is a change in medical decision making. If an order is being discontinued because it was entered in error, that may also be specified.

11. Who can write an order?

An order is typically written by a physician on staff at the hospital. In some institutions, medical students are permitted to write orders. However, the order cannot be executed until it is reviewed and signed by a physician.

12. What are the components of a medication order?

When an order is written for a medication, it is essential that the following four components are noted in the same sequence each time: [medication name] [dose] [route] [timing/schedule]. It is also possible to specify the number of times that the medication should be administered. Examples of medications orders are the following:

- Kefzol 1 g IV Q8 hrs x 3 doses.
- Vicodin/acetaminophen 5/325 mg 1-2 tabs PO Q4–6 hrs PRN for pain
- Morphine sulfate 2–4 mg IV Q2 hrs PRN for breakthrough pain

13. What are the common routes of administration?

The routes of administration and some of their common abbreviations are listed in Table 5-3. The route of administration must be specified with each medication order.

TABLE 5-3. ROUTES OF ADMINISTRATION
Mouth (PO)
Intravenous (IV)
Subcutaneous (SC/SubQ)
Intramuscular (IM)
Rectally (PR)
Topical
Inhalation
Feeding tube

14. **How is the frequency of administration specified?**
Terminology commonly used in specifying medication dosing frequency is listed in Table 5-4. Orders can also be written PRN (*pro re nata*, meaning "as needed" in Latin) and specifying a condition in which it should be administered. For example, an order that is often written is "Tylenol 325/650 mg PO Q4–6 hrs PRN for pain/fever."

TABLE 5-4. FREQUENCY OF ADMINISTRATION

QX	Every X Hours
QAM/PM	Every morning/evening
QHS	Before bed
Qshift	Every nursing shift (generally every 8 hours, but will depend on the medical center)
Daily*	Once a day
BID	Two times a day
TID	Three times a day
QID	Four times a day

**Important note:* many medical centers have forbidden the use of certain abbreviations, e.g., "QD" for daily or "QOD" for every other day, as these can be easily mistaken for one another.

15. **Provide examples of advantages and disadvantages of PRN orders.**
An advantage of a PRN order is having a standard patient care order to address common issues that arise in hospitalized patients such as nausea or itching at a site cleaned with Betadine solution. An example of a disadvantage is writing PRN pain medication for a postoperative patient who is expected to have significant pain but is unable to ask for medication until the pain is noticeable and beyond prevention. At this point, the long-term analgesic may not take effect until the patient has significant discomfort. For this reason, it may be better to initially order a regular analgesic dosing regimen for such a patient.

16. **How can the execution of an order be expedited?**
Orders written *STAT* are executed as soon as possible and are typically carried out within one hour. Orders can also be urgent or routine. *Urgent* orders are orders that should be completed by the end of a shift or that nursing staff should pay special attention to, but do not merit STAT coding. *Routine* orders are orders that should be completed daily. An example of a STAT order is a chest x-ray requisition for a patient who is desaturating. An example of a routine order is an order for morning laboratory tests (written the day before). If physicians would like a medication to be administered as soon as possible, the order is often written as *now*. For example, to provide an extra dose of Lasix, a physician may write: "Lasix 40mg IV x 1 NOW."

17. **What are the components of a diagnostic imaging order?**
Imaging orders usually involve selecting a modality and specifying the region of interest. When plain radiographs are ordered, the view must be specified. Computed tomography and magnetic resonance imaging can be done with or without contrast material and a choice must be specified. A brief pertinent history and questions to be answered must also be provided. An example of an order for a patient presenting to the emergency department with a gross deformity of the right femur is displayed in Table 5-5.

TABLE 5-5. INFORMATION NECESSARY FOR AN IMAGING ORDER	
Studies requested	Portable x-ray, anteroposterior (AP) and lateral views of right femur, hip, and knee
Pertinent history	25-year-old female with gross deformity of right femur and pain after $<$10-foot fall
Question to be answered	Evaluate for fracture

18. **Define verbal orders.**
Verbal orders are given directly to the nursing staff, either in person or over the telephone. Nurses are authorized to write down and follow through with certain orders given verbally by a resident or physician on staff at the hospital. These orders are recorded by the nurses in the medical record and eventually require a physician's signature. Orders such as these are typically given when the physician is either unable to physically write the order or in cases of emergency when orders need to be followed immediately. For example, verbal orders are extremely common during codes.

19. **Define DNR/DNI orders and code status.**
DNR/DNI is an abbreviation for "do not resuscitate, do not intubate" and refers to a patient's code status. Each patient, on admission to a hospital, should be asked about his or her desires should a medical catastrophe require the use of code with "heroic measures." These measures generally include (but may not be limited to) cardiac defibrillation, intubation with mechanical ventilation, and chest compressions. They may also include the use of vasopressors or inotropes to support circulation. Each patient may have different desires, and it is of utmost importance to determine these before any catastrophic event occurs.

A patient is considered to be *full code,* if they would like everything possible to be done in a code situation. A patient may also opt to be DNI, but not DNR, meaning they would like to be resuscitated until the point at which intubation is indicated. It is important to make sure the patient understands each of the code statuses so that he or she can make a fully informed decision. After the status is determined, it must be recorded within the medical documentation. In cases of emergency or if desires are unknown ahead of time, the default is to presume that patients are full code and would like to have everything possible done to extend their life.

DNR/DNI may be officially designated in different ways, depending on the institution and state laws. For example, in some areas variations of code status may be written as DNR-A or DNR-B.

20. **Explain sliding scale orders.**
Sliding scale orders are most commonly used in reference to insulin administration. In certain intensive care settings, the administration of electrolytes (i.e., potassium in cardiac units) may also be written in this format. These orders are written with parameters for administration of the given medication/supplement. An example follows below:

"If $3.2 < K^+ < 3.4$ give 80 mEq potassium chloride; if $3.4 < K^+ < 3.6$ give 60 mEq potassium chloride; if $3.6 < K^+ < 3.8$ give 40 mEq potassium chloride; if $3.8 < K^+ < 4.0$ give 20 mEq potassium chloride; if $K^+ > 4.0$ give no potassium"

These orders may either have special order forms to be filled out in addition to the regular order, or they may be standardized by the each institution. The term *sliding scale* is used to describe these orders because the dosage administered "slides" along the scale set forth by the written parameters.

21. Explain the process of ordering a patient diet.
Many patients will be admitted to the hospital with a provisional diet of NPO (*nil per os*, Latin for nothing orally). Patients who are expected to undergo certain imaging/studies or anesthesia/surgery will often be NPO to minimize the risk of aspiration. Theoretically, this is the default diet of every patient in the hospital, unless a physician has ordered a specific diet. However, if a patient needs to remain NPO for any reason, the most assured way to achieve that is to write an order "Patient is NPO." If a patient has a procedure the next day, "NPO after midnight" is commonly written. Once the indications for fasting are over, the physician should write for a diet. If the physician does not write for a diet, the patient will not get to eat! Several common hospital diets are displayed in Table 5-6.

TABLE 5-6. COMMON HOSPITAL DIETS

Cardiac Diet	Low Salt, Low Cholesterol
ADA diet	"Diabetic diet." Low glucose and approved by American Diabetic Association
Mechanical, soft	For patients with limitations on chewing/swallowing, generally consists of purees and jello.
Clears	Clear fluids, such as water and soup broth. Generally used in advancing the diet of postsurgical patients.
Advance as tolerated	Slowly change from patient's current diet (e.g., clears) to a regular diet. Increase diet in small portions with adequate time between feedings.
Regular diet	No limitations; the patient can eat any hospital food.

22. Discuss the difference between an electronic and a paper medical record.
Many medical centers are moving toward an electronic medical record (EMR) and are abandoning the traditional paper charts and orders. EMRs are designed to accomplish several goals. First, they allow easy access of patient information from any location. In contrast, reviewing a paper medical record requires the physical chart in hand. Second, the EMR is meant to help reduce errors in medical care. Because electronic information is typed and is usually more legible, an EMR decreases the possibility of a wrong medication or dosage being administered. However, an EMR does have some disadvantages. Specifically, it makes it easier to copy and paste previous medical records, sometimes without proper assessment. Because of the limitations in physicians' time, they may be tempted to just copy and paste from the previous day's note rather than compose a new note. This practice risks repeating information from the previous day that may no longer be up to date or may even be inaccurate. When EMRs are used, it is important to assure that each note is accurate, updated, and specific to its purpose.

23. Explain why documentation written by medical students needs an addendum.
Any information in the medical record must be reviewed by a licensed medical professional. In some institutions, medical students can write, or "scribe" notes for physicians, but they must acknowledge that a licensed physician has reviewed the content recorded in the note. The acknowledgement/addendum is typically found at the end of the medical note. An example is the following:

The above note was scribed by Jane Smith, MS4, for Dr. Jones. Dr. Jones personally obtained the complete history and physical exam. The above note was reviewed and modified as his own.

KEY POINTS: MEDICAL DOCUMENTATION AND WRITING ORDERS

1. The medical record is intended to provide a detailed account of the care that a patient receives, is essential for quality and continuity of care, and plays a significant role for billing and legal purposes.
2. A daily progress note is most commonly written in the SOAP format, which stands for Subjective, Objective, Assessment, and Plan.
3. An order is a single specific instruction to be implemented according to a patient's medical care protocol. Some orders may be executed only once, whereas others may be scheduled to occur at regular intervals.
4. When writing an order for a medication it is essential that the following four components are noted in the same sequence each time: [medication name] [dose] [route] [timing/schedule].
5. It is important to always document a patient's code status when he or she is admitted to the hospital.

CHAPTER 6

ROUNDS

Javier A. Valle

1. **What are rounds?**
   Rounds are a medical team's daily evaluation of each patient cared for on a clinical service. This includes an organized assessment of the patient's diagnoses and pathologic condition as well as a formulation of a management plan.

2. **List the different types of rounds.**
   There are various types of rounds, and they can be very different from each other. There are work rounds, teaching rounds, table rounds, and grand rounds. The attending on each service will decide on a day-to-day basis which types of rounds will occur.

3. **What are work rounds?**
   Work rounds are the most time-efficient form of rounding. They involve presenting the patient's pertinent history in a very short and efficient manner (for example, only overnight events or pertinent positive and negative aspects), reviewing the task list for each patient, and creating a plan of management for the day. The emphasis is on efficiency. These rounds are usually performed while walking around the hospital to each patient's room, discussing each patient's case outside the patient's door. After discussing the patient, the team will enter the room to discuss the plan with the patient.

4. **Describe teaching rounds.**
   Teaching rounds are significantly different from work rounds. Generally they will involve a formal and complete patient presentation, which will be followed by several teaching points. There may be a formal teaching session before/after rounding, or each patient can become an individual teaching session. Many attendings will conduct this teaching session in the Socratic method by asking the medical students a variety of questions. This is also known as "pimping." These rounds are extremely educational but can take much more time.

5. **What are table rounds?**
   Table rounds are a combination of work and teaching rounds. The team is seated around a table and discusses each patient, their interesting clinical findings, and any teaching points. These rounds do not involve walking or direct patient interaction. Patients are presented as if the team were in front of his or her door, but the team does not actually attend rounds as a whole. Instead, the senior resident and attending will "walk round" or the attending will go see the patient on his or her own.

6. **Explain the concept of grand rounds.**
   Grand rounds are usually once-weekly gatherings of everyone within a specialty, including faculty, residents, or visiting professors. During these sessions, particularly interesting patients or areas of departmental research are commonly presented. These sessions can be thought of as hospital-wide teaching rounds. Each patient presentation is developed with the intention of educating the audience on a clinical topic.

Grand rounds can also be called a different name, depending on the clinical service. For example, the surgical equivalent can be called Death and Complications (D&C) or Morbidity and Mortality (M&M). These types of rounds are generally used to discuss patients with adverse outcomes or interesting features. The goal is to spark discussion about either what went wrong and why, or what approaches would work better to avoid similar complications.

7. **What components of the medical team are present for rounds?**
The medical team is composed of several different components with a hierarchical level of authority that is displayed in Figure 6-1. The attending is at the top and has the authority for all final decisions. The senior resident is the clinical team's leader for the hands-on portion of the clinical care. He or she makes the day-to-day decisions and presents them to the attending. It is the senior resident's job to know all of the patients and to manage the residents/interns. On surgical services you may have rounds with only the senior resident. The senior resident can be viewed as an "attending in training." All non-senior residents are referred to simply as residents. However, a first-year resident is called an intern. Residents and interns have responsibility for their own patients and spend a significant amount of time working directly with medical students.

A fourth-year medical student may have the role of a sub-intern (Sub-I) or acting intern (AI) depending on the terminology of the medical institution. Sub-Is have responsibility for their own patients and present directly to the senior residents and attending. They are treated as if they were at an intern level. The third-year medical student has the least authority on the team as they are relatively new to hospital processes. Depending on the service, there may be no to several third-year medical students.

Another type of resident is a chief resident. A chief resident in medicine is one or more of the senior residents who have been chosen to take on additional clinical, teaching, and administrative responsibilities. They generally are not present on rounds with a specific medical team, but rather serve as administrative managers for the entire body of residents for each clinical service. In addition, there may be other members of the team including pharmacists, physician assistants, and nursing staff who may attend rounds with the team.

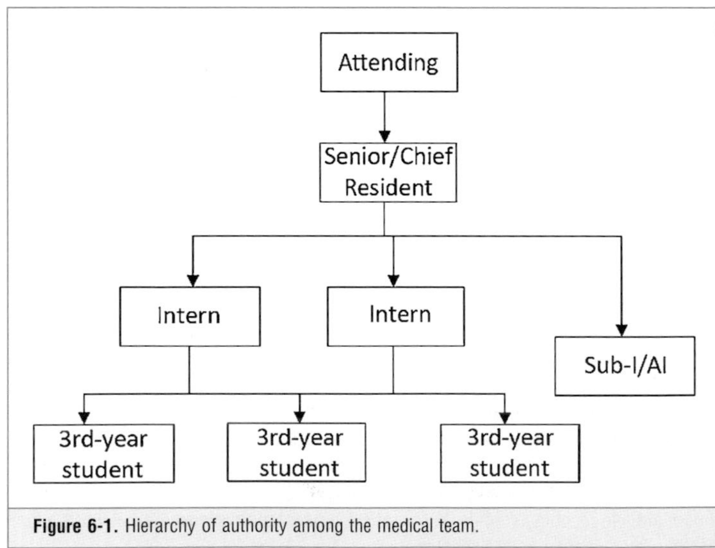

Figure 6-1. Hierarchy of authority among the medical team.

A chief resident in surgery is one of the senior residents who has additional administrative and clinical tasks in addition to their usual workload. The difference between chief residents in medicine and surgery is that surgery chief residents are not spending an additional year of residency compared with other residents as in medicine.

8. **Explain what "assigned to a patient" means.**
Medical students are assigned to a patient with interns or residents. This means that the medical student co-manages the patient with the intern or resident. The student's role often involves obtaining the history, performing the physical examination, presenting the patient, and writing daily progress notes on the patient. The medical student is also expected to stay up to date with each patient's diagnostic studies, laboratory values, and daily medications. Because medical students have fewer patients and therefore more time to spend per patient, they are considered a valuable resource by interns who manage a much larger patient load.

9. **Why do medical students work with interns/residents?**
The important reason is for patient care. Medical students are in the process of learning new clinical knowledge. Therefore, interns and residents must direct and guide a medical student's patient management. As a medical student's clinical experience accrues, interns/residents will allow for more autonomy. Ideally, as a sub-I (or AI), a medical student will manage patients on his or her own with only minor direction from the senior resident, akin to the interns.

10. **What is the relationship between an intern and a medical student?**
Interns are a valuable resource for medical students. Because of their relatively recent completion of medical school, they are able to remember what it was like to be a medical student. Thus, they can offer advice and guidance on the basis of these experiences.
Some residents can be somewhat protective of their time, but with a little bit of coaching the medical student can become a time-saving asset. If gently reminded, their teaching will enhance the medical students' education and also save them time with their daily work. For example, teaching a medical student how to write admission orders will save an intern time for each patient admitted.

11. **What kinds of things can interns teach medical students?**
Some of the main lessons are the same skills that residents are working on themselves. Some basic examples include writing admission orders, reading chest x-rays, and interpreting electrocardiograms (ECGs). This is not to say that medical students should not read about these topics on their own, but they can supplement their reading with interns' teaching time.

12. **What time do rounds start?**
The start of rounds is based on the attending's preference and can be service dependent. For example, surgery rounds tend to start early (and go quickly) because the surgeons need to get to the operating room by the time the first procedure is scheduled to begin. Medicine-oriented services such as internal medicine, pediatrics, neurology, family medicine, and psychiatry rounds tend to start later because there are no operating room procedures pending for the day. Rounds may also start earlier if the patient load is high or start later if there are only a few patients on the service. Fairly typical starting times for rounds are 5:30 to 6:30 AM for surgical rounds and 7 to 8 AM for medicine-oriented services.

13. What time do medical students need to arrive at the hospital?
As a medical student (and even as an intern), you will typically need to arrive before the start of rounds. All patients will need "pre-rounding." Initially, pre-rounding will take more time until the routine has become more natural. Generally, allow for at least 15 to 20 minutes per patient at first. Depending on the service, the amount of detail to be collected on pre-rounds will vary significantly. Surgical services typically require far less time for pre-rounding than medicine services.

14. Describe pre-rounding.
Pre-rounding occurs before rounds and involves collecting patient information such as overnight events from overnight residents or nurses, preparing to present the patient in front of the team, and formulating a medical management plan.

15. Name the different parts of pre-rounding.
The six components of pre-rounding are displayed in Table 6-1.

16. Explain the purpose of pre-rounding.
The purpose is to collect information early enough so that you have time to process the information before rounds. The next step after pre-rounding is to organize the information you have collected, both for a progress note and the presentation. Sometimes there is time to complete part of the note before rounds, or to at least skeletonize it. Either way, there should be some effort made to organize the information collected about the patient's last 24 hours so that it can be presented in a coherent fashion. Many medical students find it helpful if the resident can discuss the patient with them during pre-rounds. This way there are no surprises for the team, and the student looks well-prepared and knowledgeable during rounds.

17. Describe *skeletonizing* a note.
This is a quick process in which a scaffold is created for the daily progress note that can later be filled in. The scaffold should be consistent for each day and patient. After pre-rounding, you will have already collected several components of the note and can write them out: the subjective (S: how the patient did overnight and interval events), the objective (O: vital signs, physical examination, laboratory results, and imaging/procedures), the assessment (A), and the plan (P). Writing these out will help with preparing to present the patient.

18. What makes a good patient presentation?
A good patient presentation is organized and succinct and delivers all of the pertinent information necessary to make a decision about the plan for the day. Achieving excellence in presenting patients may take a lot of practice. An outline of how to deliver a good patient presentation is displayed in Table 6-2.

19. How does one develop the skill of presenting?
Practice is the best method for perfecting one's presentation skills. During down-time, ask a resident if they can listen to your presentation and provide feedback. You can also practice on your own. There is a significant difference between writing a note and actually verbalizing thoughts. However, that same verbalization is a skill that can be learned.

20. What kinds of presentations are there?
There are two basic kinds of presentations: full presentations and daily progress presentations. Usually the full presentation is a verbal iteration of the full medical history and physical examination and is used only for the initial presentation (i.e., the morning after a patient has been admitted). The daily progress presentation is then used for all subsequent days spent in the hospital. Within these two types of presentations, the details required will vary from attending to attending.

TABLE 6-1. COMPONENTS OF PRE-ROUNDING

1. Vital signs: read the flowsheet, record vital signs	2. Talk to the patient	3. Physical examination	4. Laboratory results	5. Check overnight orders and MAR	6. Talk to nursing staff
Tmax, Tcurrent: Highest temperature overnight, what the temperature is now. *Heart Rate:* Get the range and be sure to note outliers (e.g., an episode of supraventricular tachycardia in the middle of a night with otherwise normal sinus rhythm). *Blood pressure:* Obtain the range for systolic and diastolic and note outliers. *Respiratory rate:* Obtain the range and note outliers. *SpO_2:* Oxygen saturation. Write down the percentage, and how much oxygen the patient is getting and by what means. *Example:* RA, 2 L by NC, 60% FM. *Inputs/Outputs:* Especially important for surgical patients, and patients you are trying to diuresе. Inputs are IV fluids, PO intake, etc. Outputs are UOP, chest tube output, etc.	Did anything happen overnight? Run a quick review of systems: chest pain, nausea, vomiting, fevers, chills, night sweats, etc. The patient's nurse can be a great asset for this review. Tailor this to your patient. *Examples:* If the patient just had surgery, ask if pain is under control, etc. If the patient had an MI, pursue chest pain/shortness of breath.	Does not need to be complete, unless there is a specific need. HEENT, heart, lungs, abdomen, and extremities is usually sufficient. *Example:* You can usually spare your patients a full neurologic examination, unless they are admitted for a stroke (or if you are on the neurology service).	Check AM and PM laboratory results, and have these ready for your presentation. Keep them organized and record them sequentially. *Example:* You should have the laboratory results for every day that your patient is in-house. (You should be able to produce the exact value of the patient's hemoglobin from 5 days ago if asked.)	Look back over the orders that were written by the overnight cover team and which medications the patient received. *Examples:* STAT CBC, cultures? → Think fever workup. Did the patient develop a high temperature? CXR, ECG, troponins? → think chest pain; rule out MI. Toradol given? → Think poor pain control.	Often overlooked, nurses are a great resource. They have been with the patient all night and can tell you valuable information that you may have missed. *Examples:* Question of mild mental status changes after receiving Ambien. The patient has not had a bowel movement in 3 days and is complaining of constipation.

CBC, Complete blood count; *CXR*, chest x-ray; *ECG*, electrocardiogram; *FM*, face mask; *HEENT*, head, eyes, ears, nose, and throat; *IV*, intravenous; *MAR*, medical administration record; *MI*, myocardial infarction; *NC*, nasal cannula, *FO*, per oral; *RA*, room air; *UOP*, urine output.

TABLE 6-2. PRESENTING A PATIENT

1. Deliver the one-liner.	Truly great presentations start off with a one-line summary of who the patient is (name, age, sex, pertinent past medical history) and why they're in the hospital.	***Examples:*** Medicine: Mr. Smith is a 67-year-old man with a past medical history significant for coronary artery disease, BPH, and type II diabetes who presented yesterday for evaluation of his RLQ abdominal pain. *Surgery/ob-gyn:* Mrs. Rogers is a 43-year-old G2P1 female with a past medical history significant for diabetes, hemophilia type B, and uterine fibroids who is postoperative day 2, status-post uterine myomectomy.
2. Be confident and stay organized.	This is a medical student's chance to shine as the spotlight is on him or her during presentations. Be aware, however; attendings like to ask questions while students are in the middle of their patient presentations. These are not meant to throw students off track, but definitely can if the presenter is underprepared. If organized, a student can answer the question and go right back to where he or she left off. Using the scaffolding of the H&P/note can help one find their way if questioning leads to disorganization.	*Example:* Third-year medical student: "Mr. Stewart complained of 5/10 chest pain that radiated. . . . Attending: "Last stress test?" Third-year medical student: "Sept. 21, stress echo showed no inducible ischemia. *(Pause, collect your thoughts.)* History of present illness: patient had 5/10 chest pain that radiated to his jaw . . .[insert rest of history]."
3. Before presenting, ask questions.	Use the residents. They know the faculty and their preferences. Ask your residents about the attending: what does he or she like in the presentation?	*Example:* Short versus long? Does the attending want to know all of the social history or does he or she just want to know if the patient smokes or drinks?

BPH, Benign prostatic hyperplasia; *G2P1*, gravida 2 para 1; *H&P*, history and physical examination; *RLQ*, right lower quadrant.

21. **Explain the *full presentation.***
This is essentially a verbal review of the complete history and physical examination. However, most attendings will prefer only pertinent positive and negative points (i.e., it is unnecessary to read aloud the entire review of systems, but instead focus on what would be considered important to the patient's clinical course) in both the history and the physical examination. However, if you are unsure, it is always better to err on the side of giving too many details rather than not enough. The components of the full patient presentation are displayed in Table 6-3.

TABLE 6-3. COMPONENTS OF THE FULL AND DAILY PATIENT PRESENTATION

Initial Full Presentation	Daily Presentation
CC: Chief complaint (i.e., why the patient is in the hospital) *HPI* [history of present illness]: One-liner, followed by details. Use the PQRST framework to assess the patient's chief complaint. *Past medical/surgical history:* *Medications:* *Allergies:* *Family history:* *Social history:* *Vital signs:* *Physical examination:* *Laboratory values:* *Imaging/procedures:* *Assessment:* *Plan:*	*S: Subjective.* How the patient is feeling, what happened overnight, pertinent positive and negative aspects, additional history elicited. *O: Objective.* Your objective findings. These include: Vital signs Physical examination (usually just limited to pertinent positive and negative aspects and anything that has changed) Laboratory values (also usually just the pertinent ones) Any new imaging/procedures *A: Assessment.* Presenter's thoughts on the underlying medical process. Commit to a diagnosis as best you can. *Example:* if a 73-year-old patient comes in with left lower quadrant pain and peritoneal signs, say that she has a likely diagnosis of diverticulitis. *P: Plan.* What do you want to do for the patient? Try to formulate a unique plan and suggest it.

PQRST, Provokes, quality, radiation, severity, timing.

22. **Explain the *daily progress* presentation.**
This is the much shorter SOAP format, the same format that should be used in daily progress notes. *S* is for subjective, *O* is for objective, *A* is for assessment, and *P* is for plan. It is a simple approach and is generally the standard for conveying everything needed to be known about the patient in a short and concise manner. The important thing to remember about presentations is organization. The standardized organization is not just to help the presenter put it together, but also to help the listener interpret the information. Attendings are trained to listen and look for certain information in a specific order. It is the medical student and resident's job to convey that information in that order. The components of the daily SOAP patient presentation are shown in Table 6-3.

23. Define the chief complaint.

This is why the patient is in the hospital. It should be the answer to the first question asked:

Q: "What brings you in today?"

A: The chief complaint.

The complaint should be stated in the patient's words. In other words if the patient says "chest pain," the chief complaint should be "chest pain" and not "myocardial infarction," even if the patient has ECG changes and elevated troponin levels. The focus here is to describe the patient's symptoms, not to state the most likely diagnosis.

24. What are the components of the history of present illness?

Collecting a patient's history can sometimes be difficult, depending on the patient and historian, as they are not necessarily the same person. The key component to eliciting history is to describe the chief complaint. A good acronym for the main descriptors is PQRST (although this process is framed mainly for describing pain, it can be applied for almost any complaint):

P is for *provokes*: what provokes the issue? What makes it start, get better, worse?

Q is for *quality*: Describe it. If it is pain, is it sharp/dull/crushing? Where?

R is for *radiation*: Does it go anywhere else?

S is for *severity*: Rate it on a scale of 1 to 10

T is for *timing*: When did it start, for how long, how often?

Another key component is to always acknowledge who contributed to the history, e.g., the patient, the parents, the spouse, or the children, as each historian can provide a different variation of the information.

25. Where are the vital signs recorded?

Vital signs are recorded on flowsheets, usually kept next to the patients' rooms. Vital signs are usually recorded by the nursing staff, but at times it is advisable to take a manual pulse and measure a blood pressure if the recorded values do not seem correct. In some institutions vital signs are recorded electronically as well.

26. What is a flowsheet?

Flowsheets are the location on which a patient's information is recorded by the nursing staff. They are essentially timelines, with each flowsheet spanning a period of 24 hours over which the patient has various measurements recorded, such as vital signs, inputs and outputs, and pain scores. Flowsheets are generally located next to the patient's room, or the information may be recorded online if the hospital has an electronic medical record.

27. Where is information on a patient's medications recorded?

The medical administration record (MAR) is the prime source for medication information. The MAR can reveal the following:

- The patient's current medications and status (active, on hold, etc.)
- The scheduled dosing regimen
- The time the patient *actually received* the medication (as this can vary from the scheduled time)

Checking the MAR should always be part of morning pre-rounding. If there are some aberrant vital signs of note (e.g., blood pressure values that are too high or too low), check to see if they correlate with the administration of certain medications (e.g., when were antihypertensive medications given?).

28. Where are laboratory results posted?

This will vary from institution to institution. Hospitals with electronic medical records will have laboratory results posted online for review. However, some hospitals still use the traditional paper system. Thus, these may be in the patient's chart or written on the flowsheet.

29. What set of laboratory values are included in the daily patient presentation?

The patient presentation should include the most up-to-date set of laboratory values. At some larger institutions blood samples for morning laboratory values are theoretically supposed to be drawn at 6 AM. However, because of the sheer number of patients needing laboratory tests and blood draws, the actual timing can vary from right at 6 AM to much later. Ideally, each presentation in the morning should have the laboratory values from that morning's blood draw, as well as any other pertinent laboratory results, such as cultures that are pending or any special send-outs. Speaking generally, the most common laboratory values that will be included in any basic presentation will be a complete blood count (CBC) and basic chemistry values (known as a Chem 7 at some hospitals): sodium, potassium, chloride, CO_2, blood urea nitrogen (BUN), creatinine, and glucose. It is important to note as a medical student that blood urea nitrogen is read as "B-U-N" and never "bun."

30. Explain what comprises imaging. How should an image be presented on rounds?

Imaging is a catch-all term for studies such as chest x-rays, computed tomographic scans, magnetic resonance imaging, and even invasive procedures such as angiography (i.e., cardiac catheterization). They are tests to capture an image of some aspect of a patient. These tests are generally interpreted by radiologists, and an official report is generated. The medical student (or intern) is responsible for tracking down the final report and presenting the final impression. Sometimes the preliminary report is used if the report has not yet been finalized. On rounds, the attending should be informed of any significant findings in the imaging study.

31. Explain the role of procedures and how to present their results.

Procedures are performed every day in the hospital to garner more information about a patient and range from minimally invasive (e.g., ECG) to highly invasive (e.g., laparotomy). The role of the medical student is to find out the results of the procedure. What did the ECG show? What did the bronchoscopy show? What were the results of the enteroscopy? What did the biopsy show? Ask the resident for help regarding interpretation or read about the procedure to determine the pertinent details about the patient. Be prepared with the results during patient presentations. If possible make copies of the procedure data, such as a copy of the recent ECGs and have the copies available on rounds. Then the attending can look at them directly. In addition, medical students can help the team by tracking down study results as soon as they become available.

32. Is there a difference between the one-liner and the assessment?

These two may be similar or even the same in certain instances, but they are different at times. The assessment is a synthesis of all of the previous parts of the presentation and culminates in a diagnosis or differential diagnosis. The *one-liner* may summarize the history of the patient, but will generally not give a diagnosis. Examples of a one-liner and an assessment are displayed in Table 6-4.

TABLE 6-4. EXAMPLE OF A ONE-LINER VERSUS AN ASSESSMENT

One-Liner	Assessment
Mr. Smith is a 72-year-old male with a history of three-vessel CAD, 50 pack-year smoking history, poorly controlled diabetes (last Hgb A1C of 9.2 in January), and BPH who **presents with a 3-day history of fever and cough producing purulent sputum.**	Mr. Smith is a 72-year-old male with a history of three-vessel CAD, 50 pack-year smoking history, poorly controlled diabetes (last Hgb A1C of 9.2 in January), and BPH **who presents with a bacterial pneumonia versus COPD exacerbation.** (COPD exacerbation is more likely because . . .)

BPH, Benign prostatic hyperplasia; *CAD*, coronary artery disease; *COPD*, chronic obstructive pulmonary disease; *Hgb*, hemoglobin.

33. **What is expected from the medical student when developing the plan?**
The plan should be organized and address all of the patient's problems, ranging from the chief complaint to the patient's chronic medical issues (e.g., diabetes, anemia, or asthma) as well as in-hospital prophylaxis. Although all of these may not be worth mentioning during an initial presentation during rounds (especially basic management of chronic disease), they should be part of the note.
The medical student should be able to produce a reasonable approach to at least the initial evaluation of the chief complaint, such as which studies and laboratory tests to order.

34. **What should be excluded from the plan portion of a presentation?**
Part of the plan that goes in the note may not be relevant for presentations on rounds. Chronic medical issues should be mentioned in the one-liner but should not be discussed if they are stable and currently under optimal management. For example, using the previous patient Mr. Smith as an example, the fact that the patient is currently taking his home dose of Flomax (that he's been taking for 10 years without any complaints) is unlikely to be relevant and should be excluded. Also, prophylaxis (such as subcutaneous heparin or proton pump inhibitors for ulcer prevention) should not be included unless specifically asked for.

35. **Is there an outline for organization of the plan?**
There are two main methods for organization of the plan. Attending preference will typically dictate which is chosen. The two methods are to approach a plan by either organ system or problem. Using the patient case from above (Mr. Smith), an example is displayed in Table 6-5.

TABLE 6-5. EXAMPLE OF PROBLEM-BASED ASSESSMENT VERSUS SYSTEMS-BASED ASSESSMENT

Problem Based	Systems Based
1. COPD vs. PNA	1. Pulmonary
2. CAD	2. Cardiac
3. Diabetes	3. Endocrine

CAD, Coronary artery disease; *COPD*, chronic obstructive pulmonary disease; *PNA*, pneumonia.

Either way, this kind of organization allows each issue or organ system to be approached systematically. This organization is helpful in both conveying information to other medical professionals and also in assuring that each problem is addressed.

36. **Aside from attending preference, are there any other differences between the problem-based versus systems-based approach to the plan?**
Generally, the systems-based approach will be the approach used in intensive care units (ICUs). This is because patients in the ICU tend to be sicker with multiple organ system disease/failure and multiple problems within each organ system. This situation lends itself more to a systems-based approach, allowing one to address the organ as a whole. Patients who are not in the ICU tend to be less sick and have more simplistic (but not necessarily shorter) problems. This situation lends itself to the problem-based approach.

37. **How can one check the plan before rounds?**
The plan should be discussed with an intern or resident prior to rounds. He or she can provide feedback regarding the plan's recommendations. In addition, new information is often paged to the residents early in the morning and may sometimes be missed by medical students.

38. **What will medical students typically be asked about during rounds?**
A medical student can be expected to be asked about anything having to do with the patient. The goal of a medical student should be to know everything about his or her patients: from laboratory values to study results to allergies to why they are or are not receiving a certain medication. Because medical students have the most time, the system is such that they should be able to read about and talk to their patients the most.

Specific topics important to know are the following:

- The patient's medications: mechanism, dosage, and purpose
- The pathophysiology of the patient's medical condition
- The classic presentation of the medical condition (even if the patient does not present classically)
- Possible treatment options for the patient's medical condition
- Possible complications that may occur

39. **How can a medical student efficiently record all of a patient's data?**
The amount of information a medical student is expected to know can be daunting. Most people learn fairly quickly that their memory is not reliable enough to keep all of their patient information organized, especially once they start to provide care for more than one or two patients at a time. The solution is to be organized and use a *carding* system, which is essentially a portable filing system for each patient. An example of a patient card is displayed in Figure 6-2.

Carding systems vary with personal preference and there are various permutations that are available on the Internet or in hard copy. Asking fellow medical students or residents for a copy of one of their blank cards can be helpful. However, any good carding system should include a summary of the medical history and physical examination (H&P), the patient's medications, laboratory values, physical examination findings/vital signs, and a daily to-do list. Essential components of a carding system are described in Table 6-6.

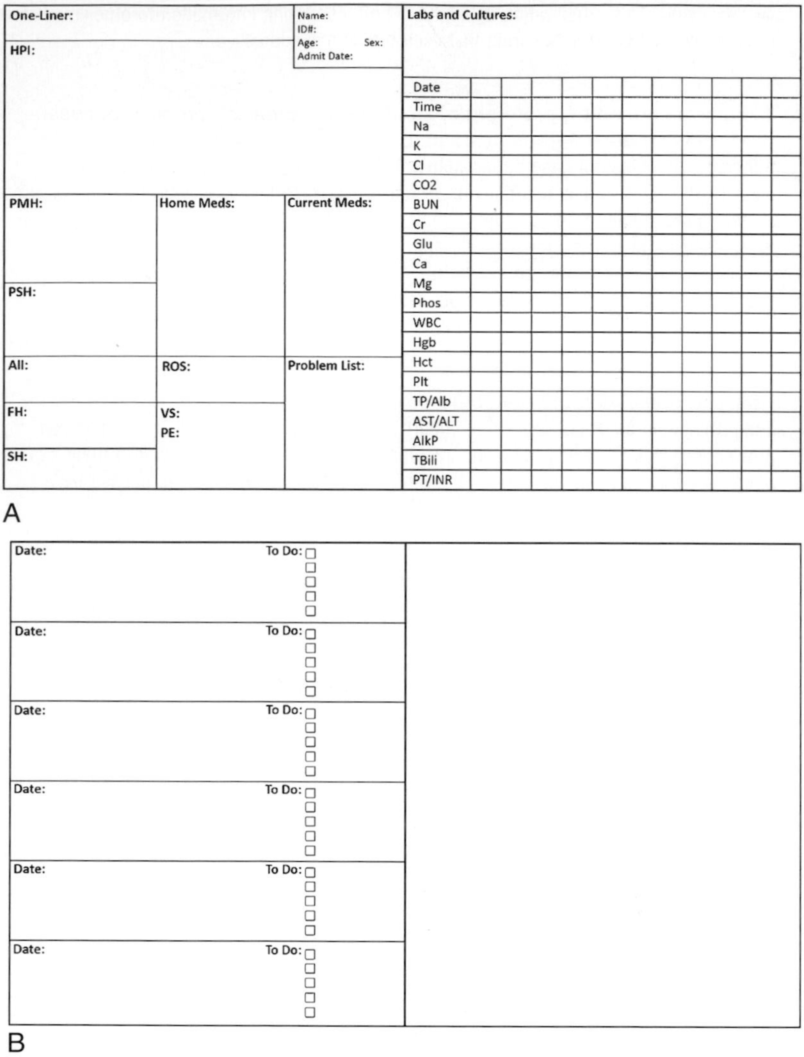

One-Liner:			Name: ID#: Age: Sex: Admit Date:
HPI:			
PMH:	Home Meds:	Current Meds:	
PSH:			
All:	ROS:	Problem List:	
FH:	VS: PE:		
SH:			

Labs and Cultures:

Date											
Time											
Na											
K											
Cl											
CO2											
BUN											
Cr											
Glu											
Ca											
Mg											
Phos											
WBC											
Hgb											
Hct											
Plt											
TP/Alb											
AST/ALT											
AlkP											
TBili											
PT/INR											

A

Date: To Do: ☐ ☐ ☐ ☐ ☐	
Date: To Do: ☐ ☐ ☐ ☐ ☐	
Date: To Do: ☐ ☐ ☐ ☐ ☐	
Date: To Do: ☐ ☐ ☐ ☐ ☐	
Date: To Do: ☐ ☐ ☐ ☐ ☐	
Date: To Do: ☐ ☐ ☐ ☐ ☐	

B

Figure 6-2. Example of a card to keep track of patient information. **A,** Front of card. **B,** Back of card.

TABLE 6-6. CARDING ESSENTIALS

1. Summary H&P (history and physical examination)	CC: chief complaint HPI: brief summary of the history of the patient's present illness (what happened, where, when, why, and how) Past medical history (PMHx) Social Hx Family Hx
2. Meds	Home medications Current medications (what was started when, at what dose, etc.)
3. Labs	A place to neatly enter laboratory values Be able to determine trends as needed *Examples:* Trending hemoglobin values to see if the patient is losing blood Monitoring daily creatinine values to watch renal function
4. Physical exam findings/ vital signs	A place to neatly enter vital signs and physical examination findings Be able to determine trends as needed *Examples:* Trending temperatures to determine how long a patient has been febrile or afebrile Trending blood pressures after administration of new antihypertensive medications Monitoring a patient's fluid status by measuring daily urine output and fluid intake
5. Daily plan and "To Do" list	Summary of the plan discussed on rounds: What there is to do for the patient that day *Examples:* Consults to call Studies to order Notes to write Laboratory tests to order

40. How can a medical student prepare for being pimped while on rounds?

Pimping is the time-honored tradition of attendings (or senior residents or fellows) that involves asking pointed questions to others on the team to test their knowledge base. There are varying styles of pimping, with attendings usually matching the difficulty level of the question to the level of training of the team member answering. Most attendings will start with medium difficulty questions to the medical student and progress in level of difficulty if the student does well. The attending may continue with harder and harder questions until the student is stumped. The important thing to remember about pimping is that the students are NOT expected to know the answer to every question. This is a chance for medical students to demonstrate their knowledge base and to demonstrate that due diligence has been performed in learning about a patient's medical care. A brief list of what to do and what not to do while being pimped is displayed in Table 6-7.

TABLE 6-7. PIMPING DOS AND DON'TS

Pimping Dos	Pimping Don'ts
DO provide an answer. Don't be afraid of getting answers wrong. Think things through and give a reasonable best guess at an answer. Attendings prefer students who at least try to think through the question. Often the point of a pimping question is for the student to get the answer wrong and then learn from that mistake.	*DO NOT answer someone else's question* until it is opened up to the rest of the group.
DO avoid saying I don't know if at all possible	*DO NOT guess randomly.* Guessing is fine, if a well thought out reason for the guess has been considered. Random guessing can lead to trouble, as the next question from the attending will be "What makes you say that?"
DO say I don't know if you are unaware of the topic and are unable to formulate a reasonable best guess. (Although it is OK to not be sure and think things out, it is NOT OK to spend time on rounds trying to talk about something that could be easily read at a later time.)	*DO NOT pimp anyone else.*
DO read about any topic that remains questionable. Attendings often bring up previous topics to ensure that medical students are doing their necessary reading.	*DO NOT make anything up or lie about data.*

KEY POINTS: ROUNDS

1. Rounds are a medical team's daily evaluation of each patient cared for on a clinical service. Rounds include an organized assessment of the patient's diagnoses and pathologic condition as well as a formulation of a management plan. There are work rounds, teaching rounds, table rounds, and grand rounds.
2. Medical students take care of patients along with interns and residents. Because students are still in the process of learning, it is essential that a physician oversees all student decisions. Interns and residents can be a valuable source of experience and information for students.
3. A good patient presentation is organized and succinct and delivers all of the pertinent information necessary to make a decision about the plan for the day. Good presentations are achieved through practice.
4. There are two main methods for organization of the plan: organ system or problem. Attending preference will typically dictate which is chosen.
5. Carding systems are an efficient method for students to keep track of patient information.
6. Students can best prepare for being pimped on rounds by knowing more about their patient than anyone else on the medical team and by reading background information on various topics that involve the patient's medical condition, symptoms, and treatments.

CHAPTER 7

CONSULTS

Derek K. Juang

1. **What is a consult?**
   Consults are often requested in the hospital when a patient develops a condition that the primary team would like assistance in handling. They are especially useful when the primary team's specialty lies in a field different from that of the problem the patient developed. For example, if a patient who was admitted to the gastroenterology service suddenly develops an arrhythmia, the primary gastroenterology team may consult the cardiology service for recommendations on treating the arrhythmia while the patient is admitted. Of course, if the patient is in an emergency situation, the primary team needs to stabilize the patient first before any consult is made.

2. **What should one know before placing a consult?**
   Medical students are often allowed to place consults. Before a consult is requested, you should be ready to (1) give a quick two- to three-sentence summary of why the patient has been admitted and the clinical course thus far, (2) have a specific question that the team is requesting a consult for, (3) know recent vital signs and current medications, (4) have a contact number or pager available, and (5) provide the patient's location and registration number.
   For example, for a gastroenterology service's patient who developed an arrhythmia, the cardiology team would be consulted and told "Hi, I have Mr. Smith, 1234567, a 45-year-old male with diabetes who presented with diverticulitis. He has been on IV fluids and antibiotics for the past 2 days, but today he developed atrial fibrillation with rapid ventricular rate on his ECG. We want to know if you could evaluate him." The cardiology team may ask about his vital signs, which antibiotics and other medications the patient is taking, and whether the patient has had any past history of cardiac illness.
   When preparing to place a consult request be sure to have the rest of the patient's information easily available. It is also important to keep in mind which service is being consulted. If you are contacting the cardiology service, it is important to have conducted a thorough cardiovascular examination and to have diagnostic test results (e.g., electrocardiogram [ECG] or echocardiogram) readily available.

3. **How is a consult requested?**
   The method for placing a consult depends on the hospital. In some hospitals, you can search for the consult team's pager number and page the consult team, or call the consult request line designated by the service. In other hospitals, you will need to fax a request to the consult team, use the tubing system to tube the request, or even simply write the order in the chart (and the nurse or clerk will call the consult team). In many hospitals, you may have to use a variety of these methods as different teams may request being contacted through different forms of communication.
   As an example, if you are paging the cardiology service regarding the previous GI patient who developed an arrhythmia, an example of the page would be "Hi, re: Smith, L (1234567). 45 yo M w/ diabetes presented w/ diverticulitis. Developed afib w/RVR, would like consult. Please call x5-5555. Thanks, John." Consult teams appreciate knowing exactly what your concern is and where they can look up more information about the patient, which is why the patient's registration number (1234567 above) is especially useful.

4. What are examples of common situations requiring a consult?
Although the primary team should, of course, attempt to diagnose and treat the problem, they should be ready to request a consult when they need help. Several common consults and who is usually contacted in those situations are listed in Table 7-1.

TABLE 7-1. COMMON CONSULTS

Consult Service	Example Situations
Cardiology	Cardiac arrhythmias such as atrial fibrillation or heart block; congestive heart failure exacerbation; myocardial ischemia/infarction
Dermatology	Unclear cause of rash or for specialized treatment for a skin condition
Endocrine	Thyroid storm; severe hypercalcemia; adrenal failure; persistent hypoglycemia
Gastroenterology	Acute gastrointestinal bleeding episodes; choledocholithiasis; cholangitis; emergency esophagogastroduodenoscopy or colonoscopy
Hematology/oncology	Any unexplained white blood cell, hemoglobin, platelet abnormalities; any newly diagnosed hematologic or oncologic malignancies
Infectious disease	Persistent fever; infection of unclear origin; treatment for rare infections
Neurology	Stroke; new focal neurologic deficit; seizure
Ophthalmology	Herpes zoster ophthalmicus; sudden loss in visual acuity
Physical therapy/occupational therapy	Evaluation of patient's physical condition and ability to take care of activities of daily living at home or at an extended care facility
Plastic surgery	Severe decubitus ulcers; nonhealing wounds; severe skin burns (caused by chemicals, toxic substances, fire, etc.)
Psychiatry	Delirium; psychosis; suicidal ideation
Pulmonary	Need for a bronchoscopy; management of severe pleural effusions
Renal	Etiology of acute renal failure; etiology of electrolyte abnormality; acute and chronic hemodialysis; hemofiltration; plasmapheresis; dialysis catheter placement
Social work	Aid if patient is unable to afford medications; needs transportation to home; need assistance regarding code status review, competency, custody, or power of attorney

5. What should be done with a consult team's recommendations?

This depends on the hospital. In many hospitals, consult teams will make recommendations to the primary team, and the primary team may choose whether or not to follow those recommendations. Because the primary team is requesting the help of the consult team, usually they will follow the consult team's recommendations. In many other hospitals, consult teams will themselves write orders for their recommendations for the patient. In all instances, close communication between the primary and consult teams is required for the patient to receive optimal care.

6. Does one need to keep calling the consult team back while a patient has a medical problem?

Usually consult teams will continue to "follow along" with the primary team. They will visit the patient daily and will offer more recommendations if necessary. When a consult team feels that the problem for which they have been contacted has been solved, they will "sign off" and will not follow the patient further unless the primary team requests more help. In addition, in some institutions the consult team may sign off if the primary team continually does not follow their recommendations for a period of a few days.

7. It is 7 PM, but the consult service says they only accept consults until 5 PM. What should be done?

In many hospitals, consult services only accept consults from 8 AM to 5 PM. If the consult is not an emergency, usually the primary team is willing to wait until the next morning before requesting a consult. It is often common courtesy to the consult team to make requests by 12 noon. Therefore, consult requests are usually the first task performed after morning rounds.

If an emergency consult is required after these hours, the physician who is on call for the specific service should be called. For example, the neurology service may only accept consults until 5 PM. However, there is always a physician on call covering the neurology patients who are currently in the hospital. For example, if a patient suddenly has a stroke, the on call neurology team should definitely see the patient.

8. Who should be consulted regarding pediatric medical problems?

There are often different consult teams for pediatric patients and adult patients. When searching for contact information for consult services, be sure to check whether there is an appropriate pediatric service available.

9. What is the role of the medical student on the consult service?

The medical student can be an integral part of the consult service. A consult service must manage both new patient consult requests and patients who are being continually followed. The medical student may have the opportunity to be the first person to go see the new consults.

10. What information should one gather while on the consult service?

While on the consult service, students should concentrate on the problem for which the primary team is requesting a consult. Medical students on the consult service should take their own complete history. Even if there are notes already left by the primary team, the pertinent positive and negative aspects may be different from what has already been investigated.

The physical examination by the consult service may be more focused than the original physical examination by the primary team. For example, when a patient is admitted to the hospital, the primary service will not typically perform a detailed eye examination (unless the patient presents with an ophthalmic problem). If the patient suddenly develops visual difficulty, the primary team will probably assess vision using a visual acuity card, whereas the consulting ophthalmology team will want to perform a more thorough examination including usage of a slit lamp.

11. What is a curbside?

Curbside refers to a primary team asking the consult team for quick advice in person or over the phone, without officially asking for a consult. For example, if a general medicine team treating a patient with diabetes wants to start a new medication for blood glucose control, they might quickly curbside the endocrine team to ask if there are any contraindications to starting the new medication. As an official consult is not requested in these instances, use of curbsides are, in general, starting to fall out of favor, for a variety of medicolegal issues. If in doubt, requesting an official consult is the best course of action.

KEY POINTS: CONSULTS

1. Consults are often requested in the hospital when a patient develops a condition that the primary team would like assistance in handling.
2. When requesting a consult make sure to have prepared a summary of the patient's presentation and medical problems, a specific question for the consulting team, recent vital signs and current medications, current patient location, and a contact phone or pager number.
3. While on the consult service, students should concentrate on the problem for which the primary team is requesting a consult. Medical students on the consult service should take their own complete history. Even if there are notes already left by the primary team, the pertinent positive and negative aspects may be different than what has already been investigated.

SURGERY

Stephen Y. Kang

CHAPTER 8

1. **Describe a typical day on a surgical rotation.**
As with other rotations, a typical day will vary from institution to institution and from service to service. Generally speaking, however, the majority of the time on a surgical rotation will be spent in the operating room (OR), in the clinic, or on ward rounds. The surgery rotation is very different from other rotations. The field is fast paced, and there is a lot of work to be done with relatively little time. Although this means that the student will have much less individual attention than a student on other rotations, this also means that the student has the opportunity to play a crucial role on the surgical team. A typical day on a surgical service is outlined in Table 8-1. Many medical schools will also have weekly lectures, during which students are typically excused from clinical and OR duties.

TABLE 8-1. SAMPLE SCHEDULE ON A SURGICAL ROTATION

5:00–5:30 AM	Pre-rounds
5:30–7:00 AM	Morning rounds
7:00–7:30 AM	Breakfast/preparation for operating room
7:30 AM–6:00 PM	Operating room
6:00 PM–?	Afternoon rounds/floor work

2. **How can one prepare for a day in the OR?**
In general, there are several tasks that should be completed before one enters the OR. First and foremost, the patient's medical record should be reviewed, including the patient's history and presenting symptoms, the clinical diagnosis, and the procedure that is scheduled to be performed. It is important to identify the presence of any pertinent physical examination findings noted in the medical record. After this review is completed, background reading should be focused on the patient's condition. The intern or resident can be a valuable resource for suggestions of appropriate reading material. Finally, the anatomical region that will be encountered during the operation should be reviewed in an anatomy atlas. Pay special attention to the nerve innervations, blood supply, and surrounding organs that may be encountered during the surgery.

3. **Describe the role of a medical student in the preoperative (preop) area.**
The preop area can be very busy with many nurses, anesthesiologists, and surgeons evaluating patients and preparing them for surgery. Ideally, enough time should be allotted for the medical student to introduce himself or herself to the patient and perform a focused history and physical examination. For example, if the patient is scheduled to undergo a carotid endarterectomy, it is important to ask about any focal neurologic deficits and, if present, about the progression of these symptoms. On examination, it is important to listen for carotid bruits. As another example, if the patient has thyroid nodules, symptoms related to hyperthyroidism or hypothyroidism should be elicited, and the physical examination should

include palpation of the thyroid. The key is to keep the evaluation focused because one will probably have only several minutes to spend with the patient.

After the evaluation is complete, double check any allergies (especially to latex or Betadine, which can be overlooked). If the patient is undergoing surgery that does not require hospital admission, it may be possible to prepare any necessary prescriptions and discharge instructions. Once these tasks are completed, the operative note can be started before the actual surgery.

4. How is an operative (op) note written?

Many prefer to skeletonize the op note before the surgical procedure begins. This involves making the outline and filling in any information that is already known. All other information can be added quickly to the note once the procedure is completed. Generally, the preop diagnosis, surgeon, and assistants are known before the start of surgery. Be warned that some surgeons do not like to complete the procedure portion of the note until after the operation, because plans may change at any time during the course of surgery. A completed sample op note is displayed in Table 8-2.

TABLE 8-2. COMPONENTS AND EXAMPLE OF AN OPERATIVE NOTE

Preoperative diagnosis	Appendicitis
Postoperative diagnosis	Appendicitis
Procedure	Laparoscopic appendectomy
Surgeon	Patel (attending)
Assistants	Schneider (HO-III), Kang (medical student)
Operative findings	Grossly inflamed, nonruptured 2-cm appendix, no abscess present
Anesthesia	General endotracheal anesthesia
IV fluids	2000 mL lactated Ringer
EBL	200 mL
Urine output	1000 mL
Drains/tubes	None
Specimens	Appendix
Complications	None
Disposition	Patient is stable and in recovery room

EBL, Estimated blood loss; *HO*, house officer; *IV*, intravenous.

5. What should be included in the operative findings section of the op note?

As a general rule of thumb, write what was observed, and this description will usually correspond with the correct findings. For example, if the patient is having a hemicolectomy for colon cancer, the medical student should think back to the surgery and describe the mass in his or her own words. The size and location of the mass should be noted. The appearance of the mass should be described. For example, if the mass is bleeding and ulcerated, this fact should be included in the op note. Next, note whether any potential metastases were found during surgery. It is important to document what was seen during the surgery. Completion of this section of the op note is difficult but becomes easier with practice. If there is any question regarding the operative findings, they should be discussed with the resident or attending.

6. **Where are the values for intravenous (IV) fluids, urine output, and estimated blood loss found?**
It is the responsibility of the anesthesiologist or nurse anesthetist to keep track of these values during the surgical procedure. Once the procedure is complete the anesthesiologist or nurse anesthetist can be asked to review the values for incorporation into the op note.

7. **How should complications be recorded in the op note?**
Asking a resident or attending for input before completing this section of the op note is always recommended, especially if an intraoperative complication occurred. This input is important because the op note may be used in future legal cases, and it is imperative that this section be recorded with extensive detail.

8. **What is proper OR attire?**
Medical students should always enter the OR in clean scrubs. Scrubs administered at another hospital or brought from home are generally not allowed. In addition, T-shirts should not be worn underneath scrub tops. Students should always wear a cap, eye goggles, mask, and shoe covers before entering the OR. Caps must completely cover all hair. Be sure to wear proper identification such as a name badge or ID card at all times.

9. **What is the first thing a medical student should do upon entering an OR?**
It is important to be aware of any sterile areas within the room, which are usually designated by green or blue towels. Typically these include the tables where the surgical kits have been laid out in preparation for the procedure. Also be aware of any staff members who are wearing sterile gloves and gowns. Anything these people touch must be sterile. It is important to be aware of these areas to avoid contamination. After locating the sterile zones, inform the nurse or technician that a medical student will be participating in the procedure. The nurse or technician will record the student's name for record purposes. If the surgical procedure has already begun, the medical students should introduce themselves to the attending and ask for permission to watch and help out. Once the medical student has been designated to scrub in on the procedure, they should either pull their gloves for the procedure or ask the scrub nurse to pull their gloves.

10. **Once the patient arrives in the OR, how can the medical student help?**
There are many things that need to happen before the operation begins, but the particular tasks may vary by operation. Students should be involved in at least some of the following tasks: transferring the patient from the gurney to the operating table, positioning the patient on the operating table, placing a Foley catheter, placing sequential compression devices, shaving the surgical area, and sterile preparation of the surgical area. Any electronic or hard copy radiologic images should be prepared for observation before the operation. These are just a few examples of tasks that medical students can perform before the procedure begins. The resident, nursing staff, or technicians can be asked regarding necessary tasks that the student can help to accomplish. Medical students should not leave to begin scrubbing until they are sure that the required preop tasks have been completed and either the resident or attending surgeon has begun scrubbing.

11. **Who are the members of the surgical team?**
In the OR, the surgical team will comprise physicians (surgeons and anesthesiologists), nurses, technicians, and medical students. The attending surgeon, resident surgeon, medical student, and scrub nurse will be in the sterile field. Some services will also have a resident fellow within the sterile field. The circulating nurse and anesthesia team will work outside of the sterile field.

12. **What are the different types of nurses encountered in the OR?**
There are two types of nurses involved in every operation. Scrub nurses organize and distribute surgical instruments during surgery. These nurses need to be sterile, and medical students should pay special attention not to contaminate them. Circulator nurses are not scrubbed in, so that they may perform tasks that involve touching nonsterile items or retrieving equipment from outside of the room.

13. What are the main points to remember when performing the surgical hand scrub?

Surgical hand scrub policies will vary from hospital to hospital. Some institutions require that the surgical team scrub for a specified time period, whereas others require a minimum number of strokes on each surface of the hands and arms. A summary table of a timed scrub with Betadine is displayed in Table 8-3. Before one begins to scrub, items such as pagers, caps, goggles, and masks should be appropriately adjusted.

Many institutions are now allowing staff and students to scrub in using an antiseptic lotion. The technique required for using the antiseptic varies by hospital. Students should pay special attention to the proper techniques for using this method.

TABLE 8-3. EXAMPLE OF SURGICAL SCRUBBING INSTRUCTIONS
1. Before beginning the surgical hand scrub, wash both hands and arms with soap and water. Arms should be washed 5 cm above the elbow.
2. Open a package of scrub wash and use the nail cleaner to clean underneath the fingernails.
3. Wet the scrub sponge and begin scrubbing fingertips, eventually working down the hands and arms and ending 5 cm above the elbow. Keep the hands elevated above the elbow at all times to allow water to drip from the hands toward the elbow. At the start of the day, this should last 10 minutes. However, if this is not the first scrub of the day, scrub for 5 minutes.
4. Rinse the iodine off of the fingertips and hands first, again allowing water to drip from the hands down the arms and off of the elbows. It is important to avoid letting water drip from the elbows toward the hands.

14. What are the main points to remember when putting on gowns and gloves?

After one completes the surgical hand scrub, it is important to avoid coming into contact with nonsterile objects and contaminating oneself. It is important to remember that at the beginning of the procedure, the nurses are very busy, so medical students should be patient while waiting to put on gowns and gloves. A summary of how to put on a gown and gloves is shown in Table 8-4.

TABLE 8-4. INSTRUCTIONS FOR HOW TO PUT ON GOWN AND GLOVES IN A STERILE FASHION
1. Back into the operating room, hold hands above the elbows allowing water to drip off of the elbows.
2. Kindly request a towel from the scrub nurse. Using one side of the towel, dry one hand and work down the arm toward the elbow. Always dry in the direction from the hands toward the elbow.
3. Using the unused side of the towel, dry the opposite hand and arm in the same fashion.
4. The scrub nurse will then hold a gown open. Place both arms through the sleeves of the gown. Even though your hands are scrubbed, do not touch the outside of the gown with bare hands. The circulator nurse will button the back of the gown.

(Continued)

TABLE 8-4. INSTRUCTIONS FOR HOW TO PUT ON GOWN AND GLOVES IN A STERILE FASHION (CONTINUED)
5. The scrub nurse will also hold a glove open. Place the hand into the glove so that the glove covers the wrist and goes over the sleeve of the gown. Once one hand is gloved, one may use that hand to help the scrub nurse hold open the glove for the opposite hand. When wearing gloves, one may now touch the gown within the sterile zone and adjust the gloves without risk of contamination. It is always recommended that two pairs of gloves be worn on each hand. Although this practice is counterintuitive, the larger glove size should be worn on the inside. For example, first put on size 7.5 gloves, then cover with size 7 gloves.
6. Each gown will have two strings to tie around the waist. These two strings are usually connected by a piece of paper near the naval. Disconnect the two strings and hand the longer string with the piece of paper to the scrub nurse. Spin in a direction so that the two strings collectively form a waistband that holds the gown snugly against your torso. Pull the string away from the scrub nurse, leaving the piece of paper in the scrub nurse's hand. Tie the two strings together.

15. **Once one is "scrubbed in," what is defined as the sterile zone?**
The sterile zone includes hands, arms, and anterior torso from the nipple line to the waist. It is important to remember that one's facial mask, goggles, and entire back, including the gown, are not sterile and therefore should not be touched by either hand. Any portion of the patient that is draped is considered sterile to the level of the tabletop. Anything below the level of the tabletop is not sterile.

16. **Describe a surgical time-out.**
The surgical *time-out* is a safety precaution to ensure that the correct operation is performed on the appropriate patient. The time-out consists of asking the patient to state his or her full name, the procedure he or she is scheduled to undergo, and if necessary, the side of the patient that will be operated upon. This occurs several times, including in the preop area and before anesthesia is administered to the patient in the OR. The surgeon conducts another time-out before an incision by verifying the same information with the other staff in the room.

17. **What kinds of questions are medical students asked in the OR?**
Unfortunately, there is no concise and all-encompassing answer to this question. In general, students should prepare for each procedure by becoming familiar with the relevant anatomy for the procedure. For example, if the patient has pancreatic cancer, relevant anatomy includes all structures that will be encountered during the surgery, as well as the approach to the pancreas. So although one should know the blood supply to the pancreas and the structures immediately surrounding the pancreas, the attending may very well ask about the different muscles that make up the abdominal wall. If the surgical approach is not obvious, the resident assigned to the case can be a valuable resource for information. The student should also read about pancreatic cancer and understand the epidemiology, risk factors, signs/symptoms, laboratory findings, pathophysiology, and treatments for this condition. Finally, the student should read about the procedure that is scheduled. The attending may ask, "What are we doing today?" It is probably not necessary to be able to recite the steps of a complicated procedure from memory, but understanding the basic plan of the operation is important.

18. **Describe the medical student's role during surgery.**
Medical students have been long referred to during surgery as "human retractors." Unfortunately, this description is somewhat true. Much of a student's time in the OR will be spent retracting, but this is an important task. The attending and residents cannot operate without proper exposure, so while retracting may be boring to some, it is important nonetheless. One should pay close attention if a resident or attending asks for the retractor because it is

highly likely that he or she wants the student to hold it but will not necessarily say so out loud. Students may also be asked to cut suture and provide suction, and sometimes they are even allowed to drive the camera during a laparoscopic procedure.

19. Describe proper use of suture scissors.
To properly hold suture scissors, place the ring finger and thumb through the loops of the suture scissors and use the index finger to stabilize the scissors. Always cut with the tips of the scissors. Medical students should never grab the suture scissors on their own. Instead, politely ask the circulator nurse for the scissors and when done place them down for the circulator nurse to pick up. Do not place the scissors back on the circulator nurse's tray.

20. Describe a method to provide suction.
Providing suction is a very important task that will allow the resident and attending to clearly see the surgical field. The challenge is finding a balance between hindering the field of view with the suction and allowing too much blood and fluid to collect before suctioning. A commonly quoted general rule of thumb is to "get in and get out" with the suction device, meaning that the area should be suctioned until clear and the device should be quickly removed until fluid begins to collect again.

21. Why should smoke from the Bovie be suctioned?
It is often helpful to follow with suction at a safe distance behind the Bovie. This helps to improve the surgical view by clearing the smoke from the field. It also helps to decrease the smell created by the Bovie's cautery. Be sure to maintain a safe distance from the Bovie.

22. What is the Bovie?
The Bovie is an electrocautery device used during surgery. It can be used to produce vessel coagulation as it cuts, significantly decreasing the amount of bleeding during surgery. When used in the CUT mode, it provides a continuous electrical current to help cut through fascia, but with a decreased ability to coagulate vessels. In the COAG mode, it uses an intermittent electrical current that provides more vessel coagulation but decreased ability to cut.

23. What are the different types of suture materials used during surgery?
Many different types of suture materials are used for various types of wound closure. Broadly speaking, suture materials are considered to be either absorbable or nonabsorbable. Absorbable sutures are temporary and are designed to be absorbed by the body after the wound has healed. Absorbable sutures are commonly used in skin closures. Nonabsorbable sutures are used when a permanent suture is required, such as in a hernia repair.

24. Describe the classification of the different sizes of suture material.
The size of the suture is related to the number before the zero in the name of the suture. The larger the number, the smaller the suture is. For example, 3-0 suture is larger than 5-0.

Large sutures are generally used to close strong tissues and are generally either size 1-0 or 0-0. Smaller sutures are generally used for routine suturing techniques within the chest and abdominal cavity. They range from largest to smallest sizes as 2-0, 3-0, and 4-0. The smallest sutures are usually used for fine surgical procedures (such as sewing together two vessels) and range from largest to smallest as 5-0, 6-0, and 7-0.

25. What are the basic ties that a medical student should learn?
Medical students should become familiar with the two-handed tie and instrument tie. A square knot tie involves one loop in the final step of the tie compared with a surgeon's knot, which has two loops.

26. Display an example of the two-handed tie.
An example of a two-handed square knot tie is displayed in Figure 8-1.

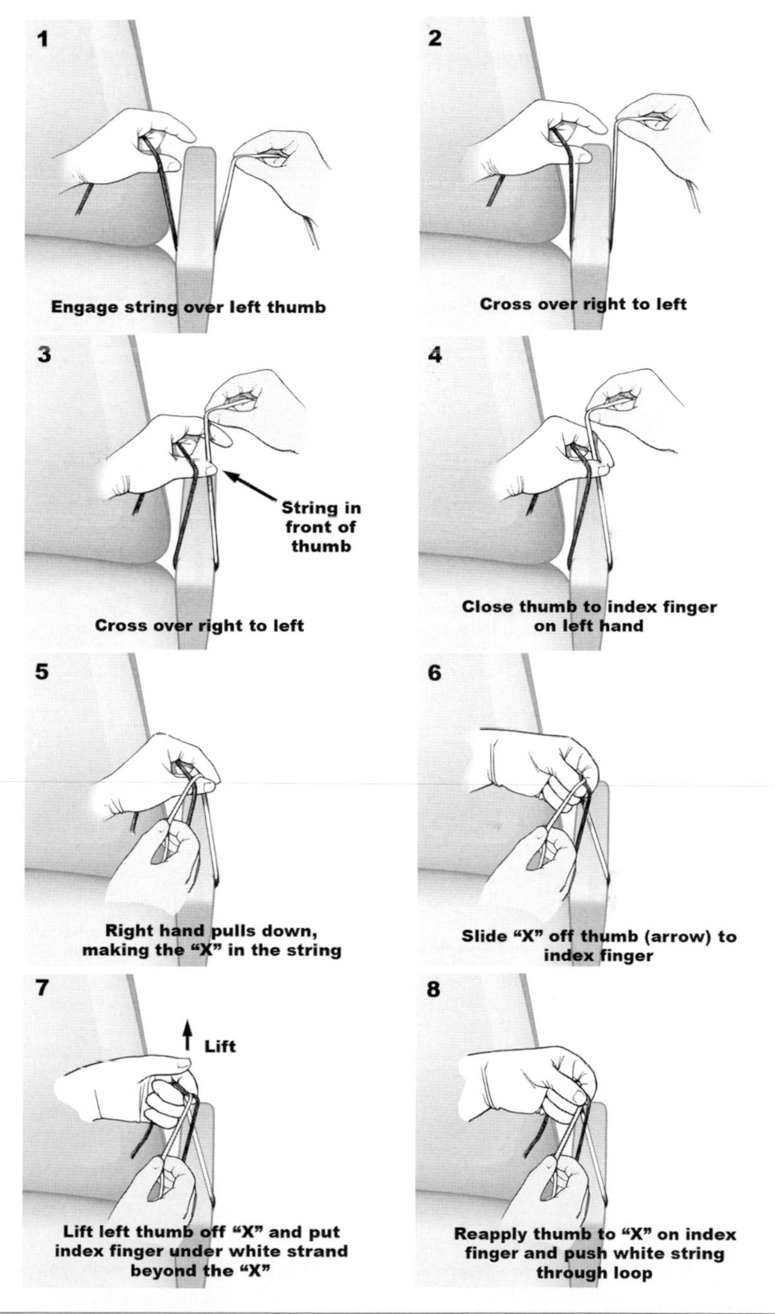

Figure 8-1. A two-handed square knot tie. (From Sherris DA, Kern EB: Essential Surgical Skills, ed 2, Philadelphia, WB Saunders, 2004, with permission.)

Continued

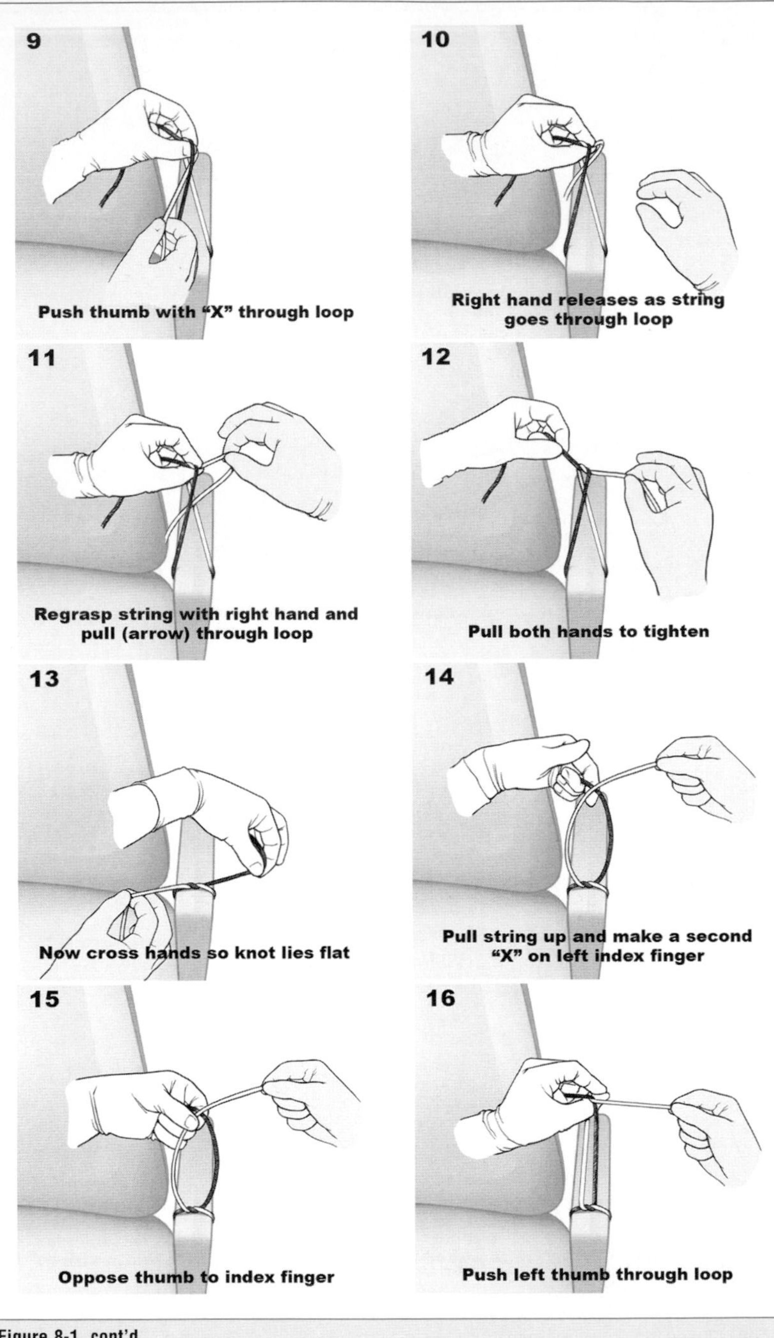

9
Push thumb with "X" through loop
10
Right hand releases as string goes through loop
11
Regrasp string with right hand and pull (arrow) through loop
12
Pull both hands to tighten
13
Now cross hands so knot lies flat
14
Pull string up and make a second "X" on left index finger
15
Oppose thumb to index finger
16
Push left thumb through loop

Figure 8-1, cont'd.

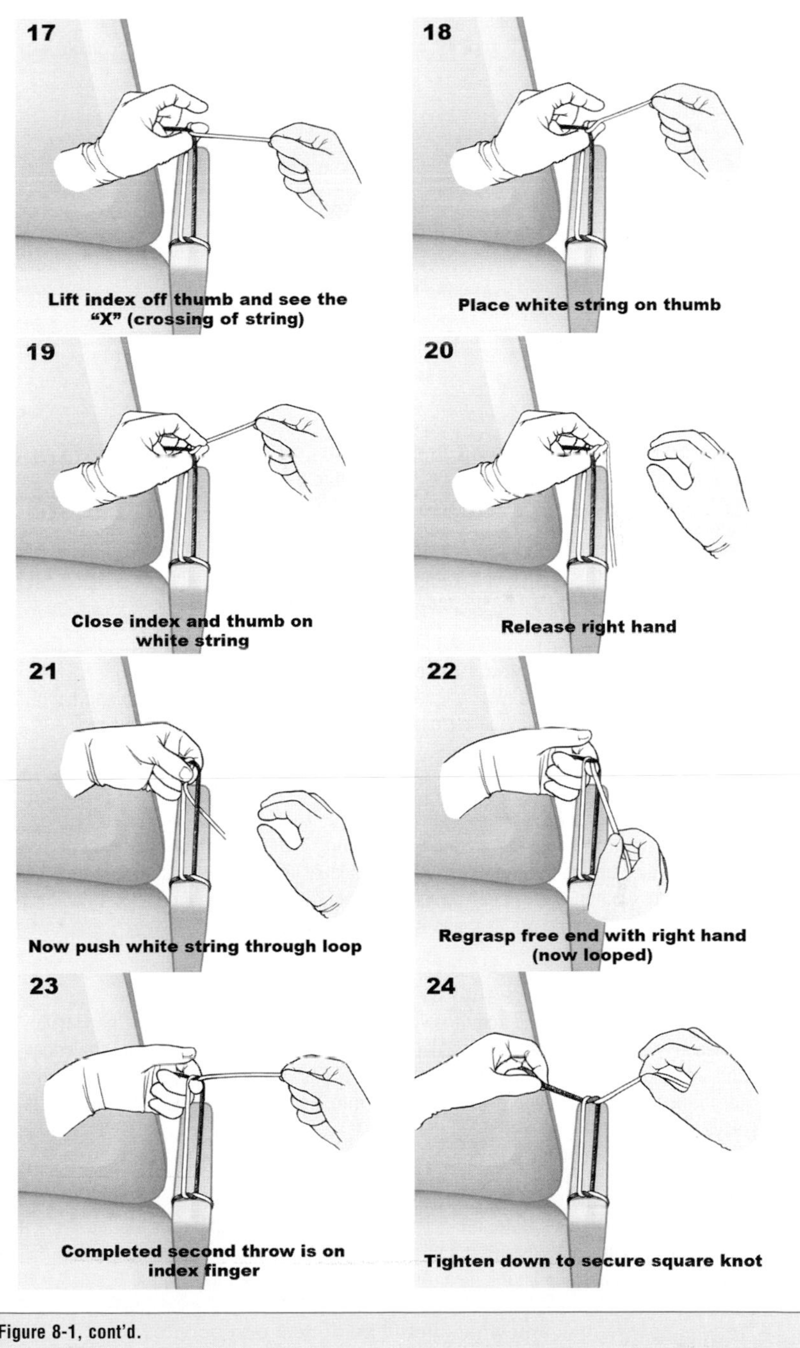

17
Lift index off thumb and see the "X" (crossing of string)
18
Place white string on thumb
19
Close index and thumb on white string
20
Release right hand
21
Now push white string through loop
22
Regrasp free end with right hand (now looped)
23
Completed second throw is on index finger
24
Tighten down to secure square knot

Figure 8-1, cont'd.

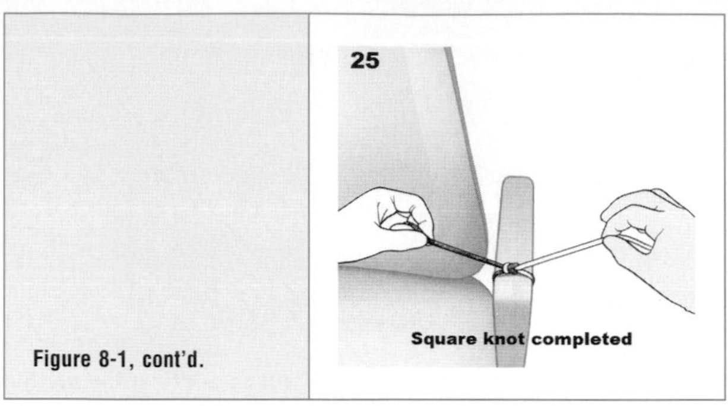

Figure 8-1, cont'd.

27. **Display an example of the instrument tie.**
An example of an instrument tie is displayed in Figure 8-2.

28. **What are the common types of suturing patterns used in the OR?**
Basic suturing patterns include simple interrupted sutures, running sutures, vertical mattress sutures, and horizontal mattress sutures.

29. **What is a simple interrupted suture?**
A simple interrupted suture is a technique that involves cutting of the suture and tying down multiple, independent knots to close the wound. An example is displayed in Figure 8-3.

30. **What is a running suture?**
A running suture, also known as a continuous suture, is different from a simple interrupted suture. Instead of cutting the suture and tying individual knots, one continuous suture is used to close the entire wound. The suture is anchored at one end of the wound and is tied at the opposite end of the wound. An example is displayed in Figure 8-4.

31. **What is a vertical mattress suture?**
The vertical mattress suture is commonly described as the suture that uses the "far-far, near-near" technique. In this suture, the needle is initially passed relatively far from the edges of the wound, approximately 4 to 8 mm. Next, the needle is passed back to the side of the wound much closer to the wound edge, approximately 1 to 2 mm, and the knot is tied. An example is displayed in Figure 8-5.

32. **What is a horizontal mattress suture?**
In the horizontal mattress suture, the needle is initially passed across the wound. Next, the needle is moved parallel to the wound approximately 4 to 8 mm and passed back to the initial side of the wound, and the knot is tied. An example is displayed in Figure 8-6.

33. **What is a needlestick and what should be done if one occurs?**
A needlestick occurs if a suture needle being used on a patient pierces the skin of anyone besides the patient. If this occurs, the surgical team should be informed immediately. Each

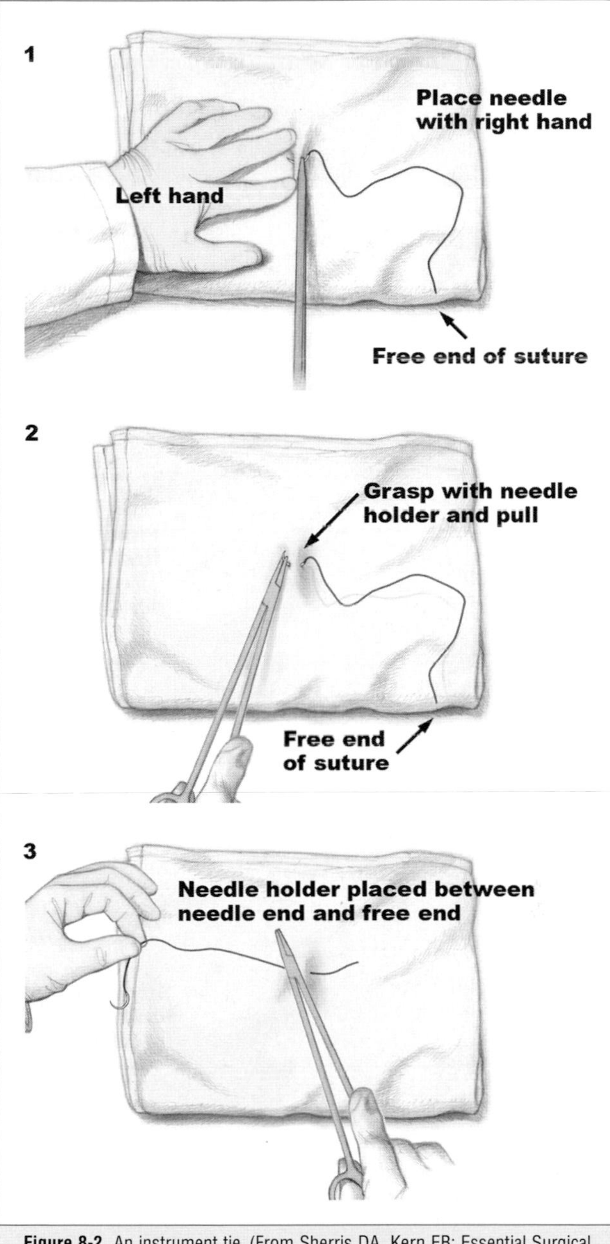
1
Place needle
with right hand
Left hand
Free end of suture
2
Grasp with needle
holder and pull
Free end
of suture
3
Needle holder placed between
needle end and free end

Figure 8-2. An instrument tie. (From Sherris DA, Kern EB: Essential Surgical Skills, ed 2, Philadelphia, WB Saunders, 2004, with permission.)

Continued

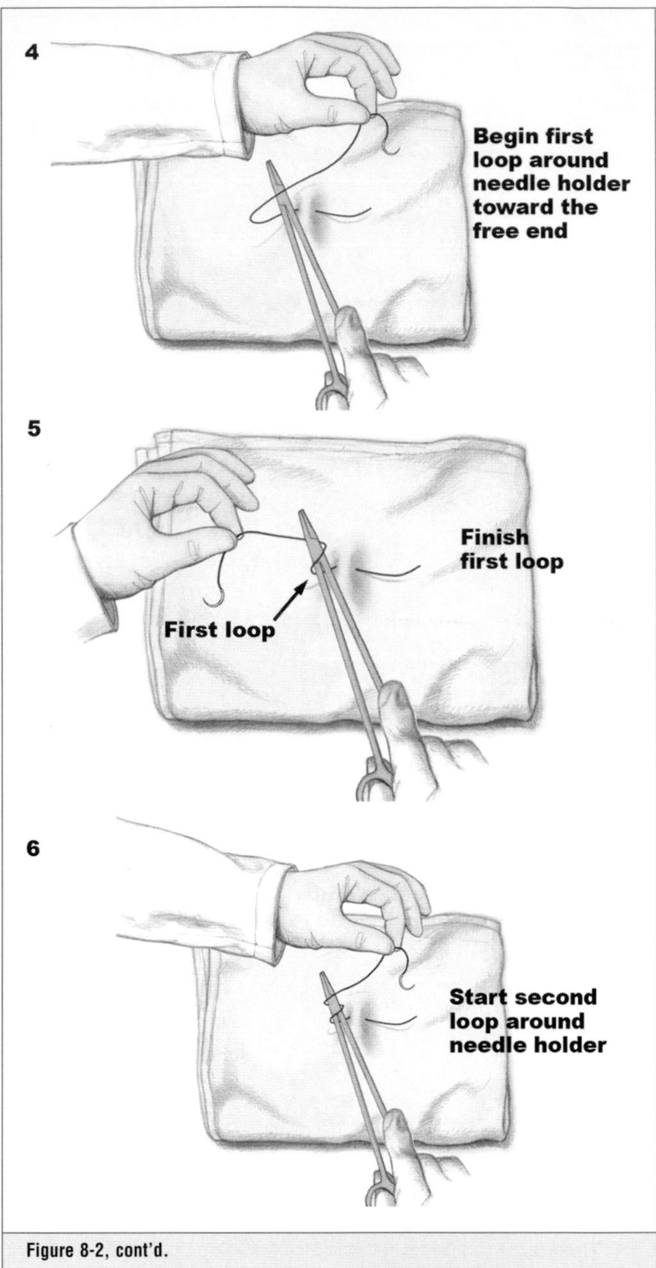
4
Begin first loop around needle holder toward the free end
5
Finish first loop
First loop
6
Start second loop around needle holder

Figure 8-2, cont'd.

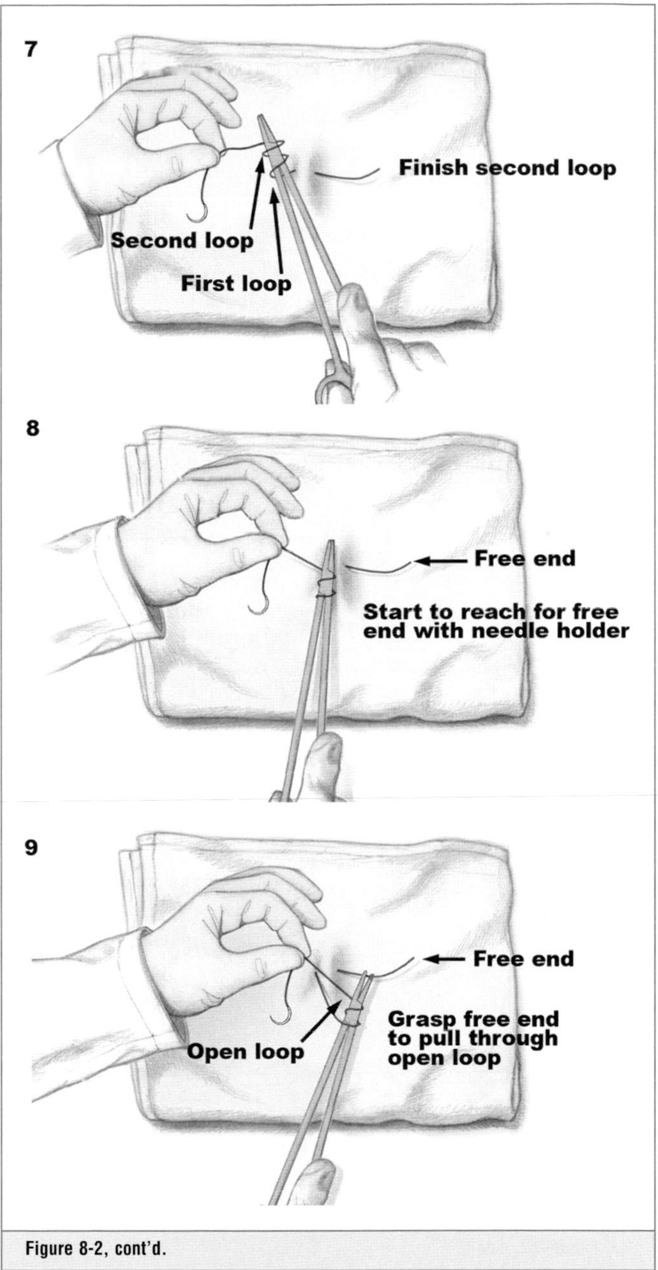

Figure 8-2, cont'd.

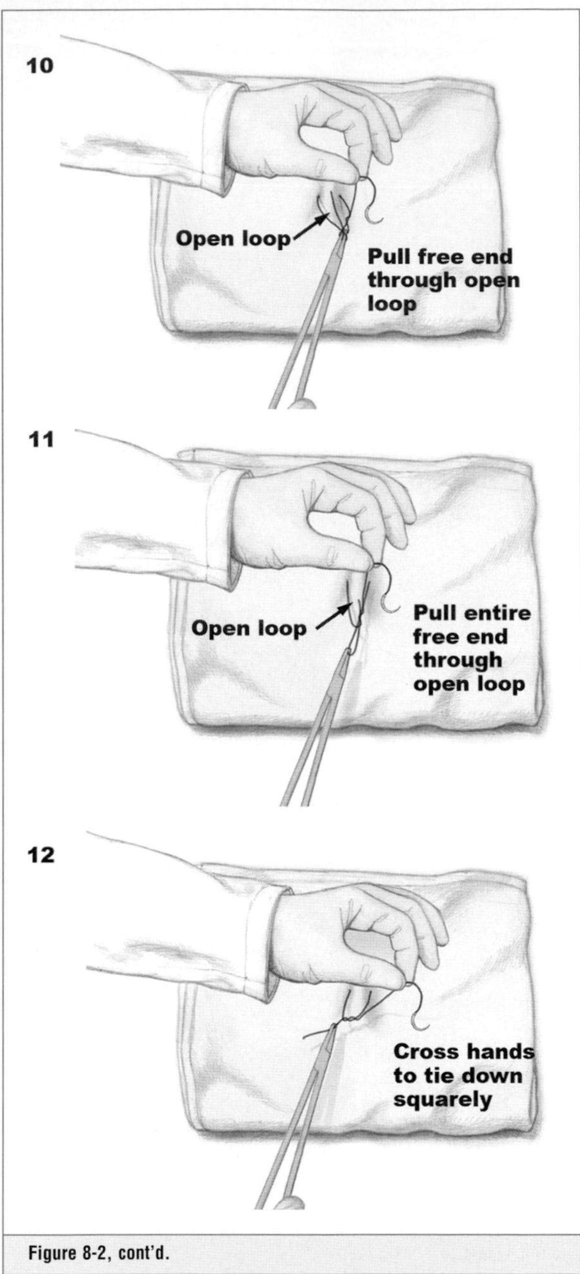

Figure 8-2, cont'd.

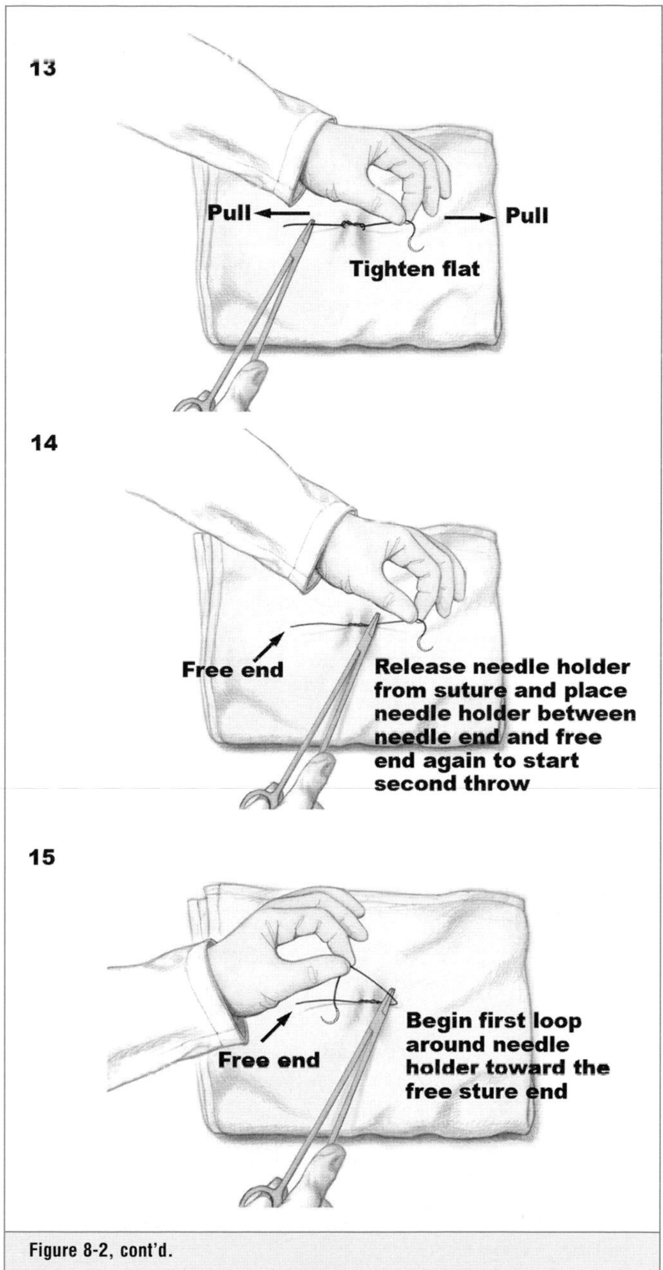
13
Pull
Pull
Tighten flat
14
Free end
Release needle holder from suture and place needle holder between needle end and free end again to start second throw
15
Free end
Begin first loop around needle holder toward the free sture end

Figure 8-2, cont'd.

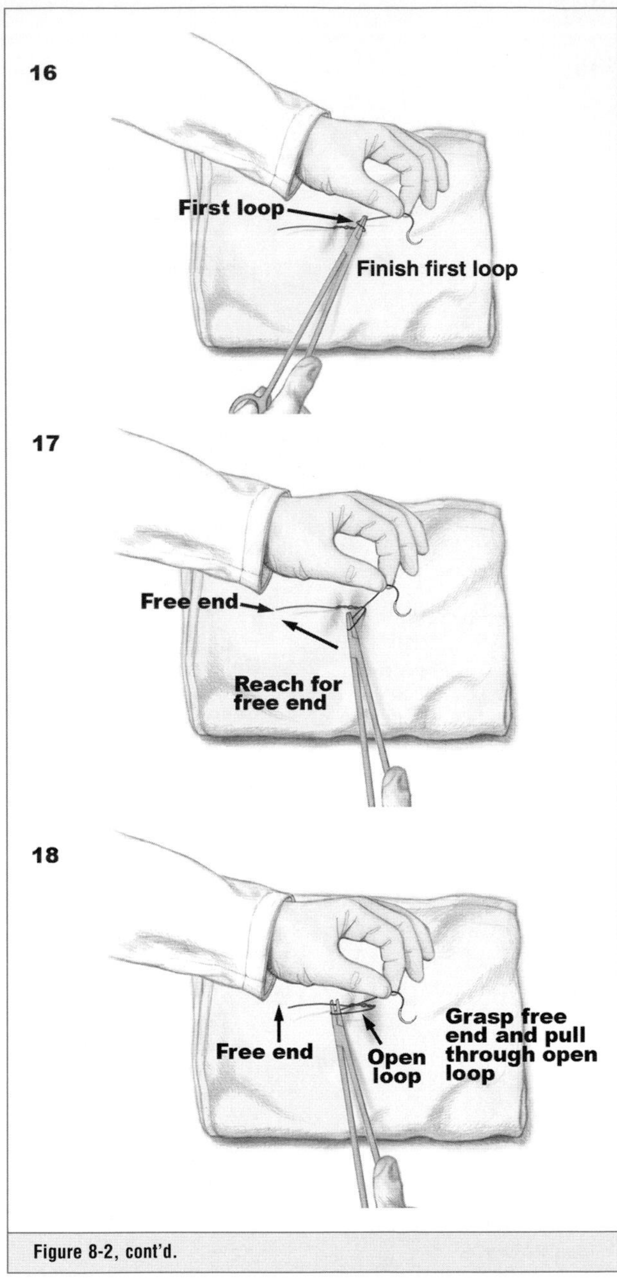

Figure 8-2, cont'd.

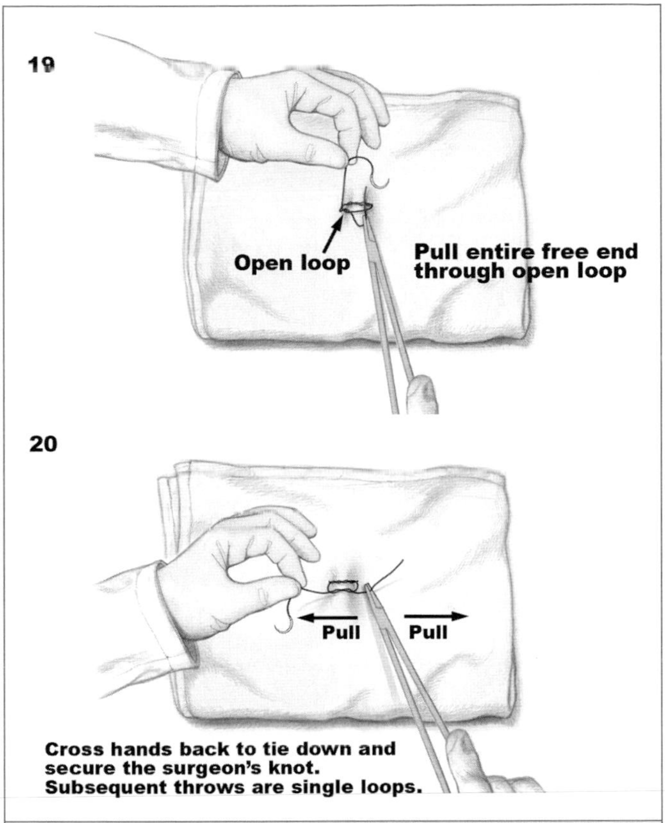

19

Open loop

Pull entire free end through open loop

20

Pull

Pull

Cross hands back to tie down and secure the surgeon's knot. Subsequent throws are single loops.

Figure 8-2, cont'd.

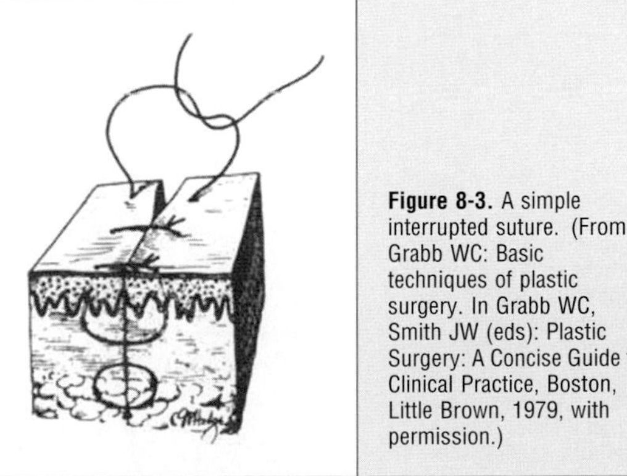

Figure 8-3. A simple interrupted suture. (From Grabb WC: Basic techniques of plastic surgery. In Grabb WC, Smith JW (eds): Plastic Surgery: A Concise Guide to Clinical Practice, Boston, Little Brown, 1979, with permission.)

Figure 8-4. A running suture. (From Grabb WC: Basic techniques of plastic surgery. In Grabb WC, Smith JW (eds): Plastic Surgery: A Concise Guide to Clinical Practice, Boston, Little Brown, 1979, with permission.)

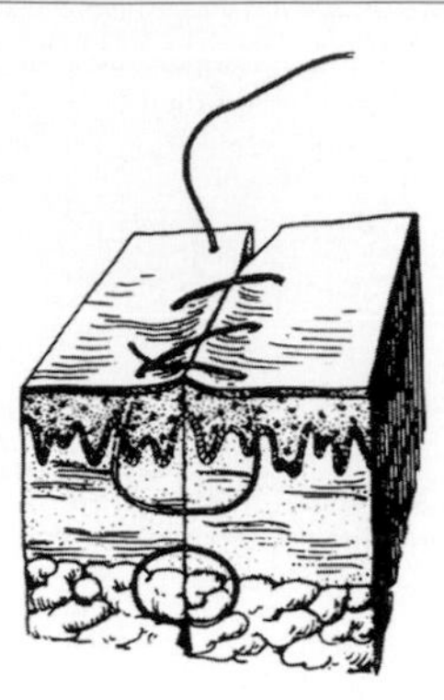

Figure 8-5. A vertical mattress suture. (From Grabb WC: Basic techniques of plastic surgery. In Grabb WC, Smith JW (eds): Plastic Surgery: A Concise Guide to Clinical Practice, Boston, Little Brown, 1979, with permission.)

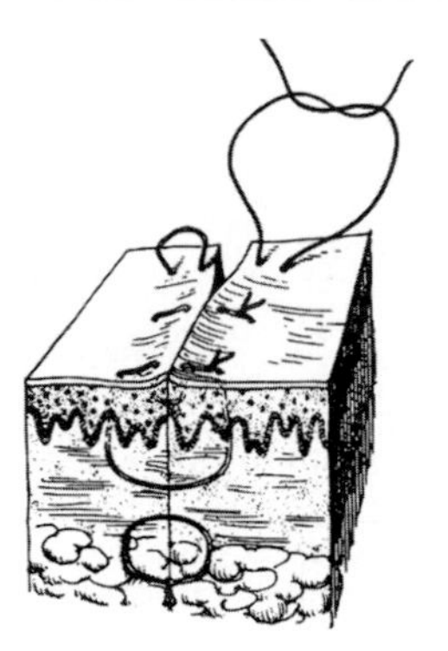

Figure 8-6. A horizontal mattress suture. (From Grabb WC: Basic techniques of plastic surgery. In Grabb WC, Smith JW (eds): Plastic Surgery: A Concise Guide to Clinical Practice, Boston, Little Brown, 1979, with permission.)

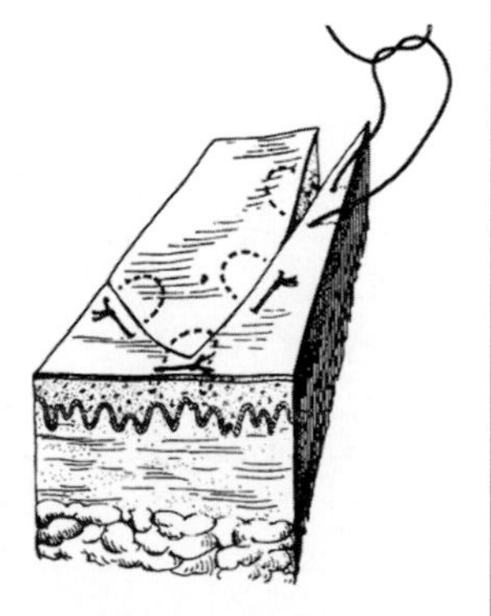

institution has a protocol for a needlestick event. Usually, this involves removing the gown and gloves and washing the area thoroughly with Betadine. It may also involve obtaining laboratory tests on the patient to rule out the transmission of communicable diseases such as HIV infection/AIDS or hepatitis and may also involve laboratory tests on the person who was stuck.

34. **What should a student do once the surgery is completed?**
Often, the attending surgeon will leave the procedure once the incision is being closed. If there is ample time and depending on the service, students may have the opportunity to suture. Students should study suturing images and be somewhat familiar with the different suture techniques. Students should pay particular attention to the subcuticular stitch. At the orientation to the rotation, you will probably be taught how to tie surgical knots. If this is not the case, you should ask an experienced medical student or a resident to teach you how to tie knots. Being prepared to suture and tie knots is a good way for a student to demonstrate his or her ability and interest in surgery. Proper suturing skills will result in increased opportunities to participate in future cases. Students can ask the OR nurses for suture and gloves to practice knot ties while at home. Make sure to practice with double gloves if that is what is done while in the OR, because suturing while wearing double gloves is significantly different from use of bare hands or single gloves.

Once the wound is closed, the student should help transfer the patient to the gurney. When the patient is wheeled back to the recovery room, this is usually a good time to complete the op note. Students can also help write admission orders at this time if necessary.

35. **Describe a subcuticular closure.**
A subcuticular closure uses the running suture technique described earlier. In the subcuticular closure, the needle and suture are placed in the dermal layer, staying in the same horizontal plane. The needle is placed through the dermal layer on one side of the wound and then is passed directly to the other side of the wound so that the suture is perpendicular to the line of wound closure. This technique results in a cleaner wound closure as the suture, if performed well, is hidden. An example is displayed in Figure 8-7.

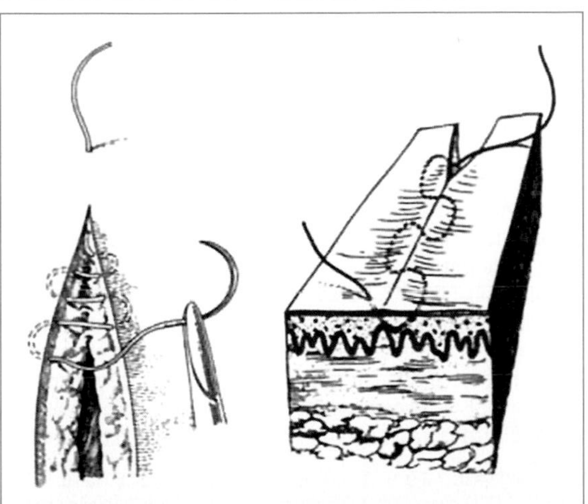

Figure 8-7. A subcuticular suture. (From Grabb WC: Basic techniques of plastic surgery. In Grabb WC, Smith JW (eds): Plastic Surgery: A Concise Guide to Clinical Practice, Boston, Little Brown, 1979, with permission.)

36. Describe surgical rounds.

The surgical team usually rounds before the day's first operation. Because the schedule is usually full of operations, the team has less time to round than teams on other services. In addition, the number of patients on a surgical service is often comparable with (if not greater than) the number on a medical service, so the pace must be increased.

Rounds are conducted as work rounds (notes, orders, and physical examinations are completed during rounds). For each patient the team will gather outside the patient's room. One person will read the board, and then the team will enter the patient's room to assess any medical changes, complete a focused physical examination, and complete any small procedures (e.g., drain removal, dressing changes, or suture removal). The assessment and plan will be discussed before the team enters the patient's room, while inside the patient's room, and/or after leaving the patient's room. Also during this process the patient's progress note, daily orders, and consult forms will simultaneously be completed by various team members (on some services medical students may be responsible for all or most of these tasks).

Depending on the service and institution, students may also be required to pre-round on their patients.

37. What is the student's role during rounds?

The student's role is to do anything that will help rounds become as efficient as possible. Specific roles will vary on the basis of institution and service. However, in general, students should be able to change dressings, remove staples, and read the board. Depending on the services, students may be expected to pre-round, present, and/or write progress notes for patients on their service.

38. How should a student present a patient on surgical rounds?

Student presentations should be short and to the point. As a general rule of thumb your presentation should consist of a brief one-line summary of the patient followed by events that occurred overnight. For example, "Mr. Jones is a 25-year-old gentleman admitted for appendicitis who is post-op day #1 from a laparoscopic appendectomy and had no problems overnight." Next, the student should read the board.

39. What does it mean to *read the board*?

The *board* refers to the flow board on which the nurses record vital signs and other important information. Unless told otherwise, the board should be read as follows: Tmax (maximum temperature over past 24 hours), Tcurrent (most recent recorded temperature), heart rate, respiratory rate, blood pressure, O_2 saturation. If the patient is receiving ventilatory support, ventilatory settings should be read in the following order: type of ventilatory support, tidal volume, rate, fraction of inspired O_2 (FIO_2), and pressure support or positive end-expiratory pressure. If the patient has central venous pressure, this should be stated after the ventilator settings. Inputs and outputs (I/Os) are then stated for the past 24 hours, followed by the urine output from the last three shifts (starting with the most recent and going back in time). Any other outputs should then be stated, such as from a colostomy or nasogastric tube. Next, any type of IV fluids or total parental nutrition the patient is receiving should be stated. Finally, read the most recent chemsticks (glucose monitoring), laboratory values, and the medications the patient is receiving. Be aware that some teams may want the board read in different fashion. However, this is a good comprehensive general outline. A summarized outline with abbreviations is displayed in Table 8-5. An example of reading the board follows:

Example: Spoken: "[One-liner] Vitals: 98.9, 97.2, 55 to 65, 14, 120 to 130 over 60 to 70, 98% on 2L nasal cannula, 24 hour I's and O's: 1700 over 2500, urine output 500 going back 600 going back 700."
Translation: "Vitals are: maximum temperature 98.9, current temperature is 97.2, heart rate ranged from 55 to 65, respiratory rate is 14, blood pressure ranges from 120 to130 over 60 to 70, patient is saturating to 98% breathing 2 liters of O_2 by nasal cannula. The patient's inputs and outputs over the past 24 hours total 1700 in and 2500 out. Urine output over the past 3 shifts is 500 mL (most recent shift), 600 mL, and 700 mL."

TABLE 8-5. SUMMARIZED OUTLINE FOR READING THE BOARD
Temperature maximum and current
Heart rate
Respiratory rate
Blood pressure
O_2 saturation on room air/nasal canula, etc.
Ventilator settings
Type
Tidal volume
Rate
FIO_2
Pressure support/PEEP
Central venous pressure
Inputs/Outputs: total for past 24 hours
Urine output for past 3 shifts
Other outputs (NG tube, etc.)
Fluids or parental nutrition
Chemsticks
FIO_2, Fraction of inspired O_2; *NG*, nasogastric; *PEEP*, positive end-expiratory pressure.

40. Should medical students change dressings during pre-rounds or during team rounds?
This is a very team-dependent preference. Some want the dressings examined and changed during pre-rounds, whereas others will defer dressing changes until team rounds. As a general rule, a student should not remove a dressing if he or she is unsure whether the dressing needs to be changed. This comment especially applies to the patient's first dressing change. Students should avoid removing a dressing before postoperative day two unless told otherwise.

41. What should medical students carry in their pockets during rounds?
Students should have the following items during rounds: 4 × 4 pads, Kerlix rolls, tape, trauma scissors, pen, penlight, and a stethoscope. Wound care accessories will depend on the specific service. The student should try to have all wound care supplies in his or her pockets at all times during rounds. If the team uses a cart to carry supplies during rounds, the student should make sure that the cart is fully stocked every morning before rounds begin.

42. How is a progress note written on a surgical service?
A surgery progress note is written in SOAP format. This consists of *s*ubjective information, *o*bjective information, *a*ssessment, and *p*lan. The surgery note should be brief and is usually much shorter than a medicine note. A description and example of a SOAP note is displayed in Table 8-6.

TABLE 8-6. DESCRIPTION AND EXAMPLE OF A SOAP NOTE

	Description	Example
Subjective	Include all information obtained from the patient such as pain control, presence or absence of flatus/bowel movements, etc. Also include issues that occurred overnight.	Patient notes minor pain around incision site. Otherwise, feels "fine" and has no additional complaints. Is ambulating and urinating without difficulty. No nausea, vomiting. No bowel movement but had flatus.
Objective	Include the information obtained from the flow board, followed by pertinent physical examination findings and the latest laboratory tests and studies.	Tmax: 99.7, Tcurrent: 99.3, HR: 78, RR: 16, BP: 124/80, O2 sat 95% on room air. I/O: 2300 mL/2400 mL over past 24 hours. Urine: 850, 750, 800 past 3 shifts. Physical exam: General: Appears well and in no distress. A/O × 3. CV: RRR, normal S1 and S2, without murmurs, rubs, gallops. Pulm: Clear to auscultation bilaterally. Abdomen: Soft, nontender, nondistended. + Bowel sounds in all 4 quadrants. No hepatosplenomegaly. Wound is clean, dry, and intact with no drainage or erythema. Labs/studies: No new labs or studies.
Assessment	Include a quick summary of the patient including age, sex, diagnosis, procedure, postoperative day, and an assessment of the patient's condition and progress	Mr. Johnson is a 25-year-old gentleman who is POD #2 s/p laparoscopic appendectomy. He is recovering without complications.
Plan	Include the team's plan, in numerical order.	1. Advance diet to clears. 2. Continue Ancef 500 mg Q 8 hours. 3. Continue to encourage ambulation and usage of incentive spirometer.

A/O, Alert and oriented; *BP,* blood pressure; *CV,* cardiovascular; *HR,* heart rate; *I/O,* input/output; *O2 sat,* oxygen saturation; *POD,* postoperative day; *RR,* respiratory rate; *RRR,* regular rate and rhythm; *s/p,* status post; *Tcurrent,* latest recorded temperature; *Tmax,* maximum temperature over the past 24 hours.

43. What types of patients are seen in the surgery clinic?

Patients seen in the surgery clinic can be broadly divided into two categories. On one hand, surgeons will see postoperative patients in the clinic to ensure that the patient is recovering from surgery appropriately. On the other hand, surgeons will also evaluate patients with a variety of medical conditions to determine whether the patient is a suitable surgical candidate and whether the patient will benefit from a surgical procedure.

44. **How is clinic on a surgical service different from that on nonsurgical services?**
Surgery clinic is a unique experience that is much different from outpatient clinics in medicine, pediatrics, or any other primary care specialty. For example, a family medicine physician will see a patient, evaluate the chief complaint and develop a differential diagnosis with the aim of determining a specific diagnosis. On the other hand, in surgery clinic, the majority of patients are referred by other physicians who have already performed an initial evaluation and deemed the patient as a possible candidate for surgical intervention. The surgeon's job is to determine whether the patient is a suitable surgical candidate and whether the patient will benefit from a surgical procedure. For example, a patient with transient ischemic attacks due to carotid artery stenosis will present to a primary care physician (PCP). The PCP will rule out other nonsurgical causes of the transient ischemic attacks and refer the patient to a vascular surgeon. The surgeon will then evaluate this patient in clinic and perform laboratory tests and studies to aid in determining whether the patient will benefit from surgery. The surgeon often must weigh the pros and cons of surgery versus nonsurgical management of the patient's condition. For example, an 85-year old man with coronary artery disease and prostate cancer will be managed much differently than the relatively healthy 50-year-old man with prostate cancer of the same stage.

45. **How can a student be successful in surgery clinic?**
The student should learn to efficiently search the medical record for information pertinent to the patient's surgical condition. Many patients will have laboratory tests and studies performed before being evaluated by the surgeon. Another physician has already evaluated the patient before evaluation in surgery clinic. The student should organize and be able to concisely present all of the work-up that has been performed on a patient before the referral to the surgeon in addition to the information obtained by his or her own history and physical examination.

KEY POINTS: SURGERY

1. Students on a surgical service will spend the majority of time in the operating room. Surgical services are fast paced owing to the amount of work that must be accomplished within a limited timeframe. Although this means that the student will have much less individual attention compared with a student on other rotations, this also means that the student has the opportunity to play a crucial role on the surgical team.
2. To prepare for a day in the operating room, review the patient's medical record, identify any pertinent history or physical examination findings, and perform background reading on the patient's medical condition and the procedure. Be sure to pay special attention to the relevant anatomy.
3. Before surgery, medical students should introduce themselves to the patient in the preoperative holding area. If time allows, perform a focused history and physical examination.
4. Always wear clean scrubs in the operating room. T-shirts should not be worn underneath scrub tops. Be sure to wear proper identification, a cap, eye goggles, a mask, and shoe covers before entering the operating room.
5. After completing the surgical hand scrub, avoid coming into contact with nonsterile objects and contaminating oneself.
6. Patients visit outpatient surgery clinics typically for follow-up visits from prior surgery or for assessment to determine whether they are appropriate candidates for surgery.

CHAPTER 9

INTENSIVE CARE UNIT

Derek K. Juang and Mitesh S. Patel

1. **What is the intensive care unit (ICU)?**
The ICU is a specialized area of the hospital designated for patients who are critically ill and may require increased monitoring, hemodynamic support, or airway support. One of the major differences in the ICU is that the nurse-to-patient ratio is higher (usually 1:2). In addition, *intensivists*, who can provide care for patients, are available. There are many different types of ICUs, and each ICU is equipped to handle various types of patients. The ICU is often referred to as the *unit*. While naming of the ICUs is not standardized, Table 9-1 shows some commonly used acronyms:

TABLE 9-1. TYPES OF INTENSIVE CARE UNITS

SICU	Surgical intensive care unit
CCU	Coronary care unit
NICU	Neonatal intensive care unit
NICU	Neuro intensive care unit
MICU	Medicine intensive care unit
CCMU	Critical care medicine unit
TICU	Trauma intensive care unit
PICU	Pediatric intensive care unit
BICU	Burn intensive care unit

2. **How are patients admitted to the ICU?**
Patients can be admitted to the ICU from anywhere within the hospital as well as directly from outside transfers. If the emergency medicine physicians feel that the patient may need intensive monitoring or hemodynamic support, they may request that a patient be directly admitted to the ICU. In addition, after certain procedures such as cardiac catheterization or surgery, a patient may be sent first to the ICU for intensive care and monitoring. If the medical condition of a patient on the general medicine or surgery floor deteriorates, that patient may be transferred to the ICU for more intensive evaluation and management. Patients requiring continued mechanical ventilator support are often cared for in the ICU.

3. **How are the monitoring and frequency of care in the ICU different from those on an inpatient floor?**
Patient monitoring is increased in the ICU. On the general floor, patient vital signs may be checked by nurses every 2 to 6 hours. In the ICU, the frequency of monitoring by nurses can range from every hour to as often as every 15 minutes, depending on the severity of illness.

All patients in the ICU are in a "monitored bed," usually meaning that they are constantly connected to an electrocardiogram monitor, pulse oxygenation monitor, and blood pressure cuff. Sometimes more invasive forms of monitoring may be used in the ICU. Instead of a blood pressure cuff, which measures blood pressure at intermittent intervals, an arterial line may be used for continuous blood pressure monitoring. In addition, other invasive monitoring can take place in the ICU, such as central venous pressure, cardiac output, and systemic vascular resistance.

4. **What is the difference in number of staff per patient in the ICU compared with that on an inpatient floor?**
The number of staff per patient is increased in the ICU. On an inpatient floor a nurse may take care of 4 to 6 patients on average, whereas in the ICU the nurse-to-patient ratio is usually 1:2 or less. In addition, other critical support staff, such as the respiratory therapists, are readily available in the ICU.

5. **Who directs care of patients in the ICU?**
In medicine ICUs, critical care physicians direct care of the patients. These attendings are usually trained in pulmonary medicine or anesthesia and have completed additional training (fellowship) in critical care medicine. In other subspecialty ICUs such as the surgical ICU, trauma ICU, or cardiac care unit, subspecialty attendings will direct the care of patients.

6. **How does the staff in the ICU differ from that on other services?**
The nursing staff in an ICU may consist of registered nurses who are similar to the floor nurses. However, many nurses either have special ICU training or have obtained certification in critical care.

7. **How does a medical student's role change with patients in the ICU?**
Patients in the ICU are more ill and require increased monitoring by both nurses and physicians. Because these patients' illnesses require more attention, medical students should check on these patients more often. In addition, laboratory results are usually obtained first for ICU patients. Therefore, medical students should check on laboratory values for ICU patients first. Medical students should be very wary about infection control and should wear gloves when indicated. Some patients in the ICU (as well as those on the general floor) may be on contact precautions, requiring the use of gowns inside their room.

8. **How does an admission history and physical (H&P) differ for ICU patients?**
ICU patients' medical conditions are more severe, and, therefore, admission histories and physical examinations tend to be complex and require more attention to detail. Many patients who are admitted to ICUs may not be able to provide their history; thus this information is often gathered from other sources including family, friends, paramedics, and other health care providers. The source(s) of information should always be recorded. The information gathered should not only contain the primary reason that brought the patient to seek medical care in the first place but also include a detailed description of the events that led to a deterioration in his or her medical condition to warrant ICU management. In the physical examination, it is important to conduct a full neurologic examination and document it in the note. Finally, as with all patients, the code status should be confirmed and clearly stated in the admission H&P and recorded in the order set by the admitting physician.

9. **How is the plan recorded and presented for ICU patients?**
For floor patients, the plan is most commonly presented in a problem-based manner. However, for patients in the ICU, the plan is usually recorded and presented by systems. Because of the increased complexity of the conditions of ICU patients, presenting patients in this manner helps ensure that all problems are addressed. Usually, the systems included (with common

abbreviations) are neurology (Neuro), cardiovascular (Cardio/CV), pulmonary (Pulm), gastrointestinal (GI), renal, infectious disease (ID), fluids/electrolytes/nutrition (FEN), hematology (Heme), and prophylaxis (Prophy). Neurology, cardiology, or pulmonary are often first on the list, followed next by the system with the most pressing issues.

10. **How does the presentation of an ICU patient differ from that of a floor patient?**
Presentation of ICU patients often involves significantly more information than that of a floor patient. Therefore, it is important to be succinct but complete. These presentations are often difficult for medical students at the beginning of their clinical rotations, because they require the student to sift through a lot of information to determine the relevant points to present. The best advice may be to practice the presentation beforehand and keep in mind the general order of presentations: (1) events over the past 24 hours; (2) subjective information from the patient (if available); (3) objective data presentation, including pertinent physical examination findings; (4) assessment; and (5) plan by systems.

11. **What are the different modes of mechanical ventilation?**
Many patients in ICUs require intubation so that a mechanical ventilator can control the patient's breathing. Although there are several different methods of ventilation, the most common approaches are assisted control, synchronized intermittent mandatory ventilation, and pressure support ventilation. One important tip is that respiratory therapists are quite familiar with these machines and their settings and are a great resource for students to learn from.

12. **What is assisted control (AC) ventilation?**
This is usually the initial mode used for patients who require ventilation. In this mode, a minimum number of breaths per minute are set. The machine senses whether the patient tries to initiate a breath. If the patient initiates a breath, the machine helps deliver a set tidal volume. If the patient does not initiate a breath, the ventilator delivers a breath at the set rate per minute. In this setting, all breaths are delivered by the ventilator.

13. **What is synchronized intermittent mandatory ventilation (SIMV)?**
In this mode, a minimum number of breaths per minute are set, just as in AC ventilation. However, when a patient initiates a breath, the machine does not deliver a preset volume. If the machine does not sense a spontaneous breath from the patient, the machine will deliver a breath in synchrony with the patient's breathing rhythm.

14. **What is pressure support ventilation (PSV)?**
This ventilation mode is typically used when one is trying to wean a patient off the ventilator. When a patient initiates a breath, pressure is delivered to assist the patient's breathing. This mode does not deliver any breaths on its own.

15. **What are the various settings for mechanical ventilation?**
Aside from setting a ventilation mode, the rate, tidal volume, fraction of inspired oxygen (FIO_2), and positive end-expiratory pressure (PEEP) need to be set. The rate determines the minimum number of breaths a patient will receive per minute. The tidal volume refers to the volume of air given for each breath. The FIO_2 refers to the percentage of oxygen delivered with each breath. PEEP is sometimes added to prevent the alveoli from collapsing (atelectasis) at the end of each breath.

16. **What parameters should be changed if the patient is retaining or blowing off too much CO_2?**
The respiratory rate and the tidal volume are the first parameters that should be adjusted.

17. How does a patient get taken off a ventilator?

This process of taking a patient off a ventilator is usually referred to as *weaning.* When determining whether a patient may be ready to be weaned off a ventilator, physicians will estimate the patient's ability to generate sufficient inspiratory force to allow proper oxygenation and ventilation. The patient will also need to be able to support his or her oxygenation with less than 50% FIO_2, because without mechanical ventilation this much oxygen support is unreliable. The patient is also assessed to be sure he or she is hemodynamically stable and whether mental and neuromuscular status is appropriate with minimal or no sedation.

Weaning parameters are often used to help physicians determine whether a patient is ready. A common set of weaning parameters is listed in Table 9-2.

TABLE 9-2. COMMON WEANING PARAMETERS
Respiratory rate <25 breaths per minute
Tidal volume >5 mL/kg
Vital capacity >10 mL/kg
Minute ventilation <10 L/min
PaO_2/FIO_2 >200
Shunt (Qs/Qt) <20%
Negative inspiratory force (NIF) <−25 cm H_2O
Respiratory rate/tidal volume <105 or <130 in elderly patients

FIO_2, Fraction of inspired oxygen; *PaO_2,* partial pressure of arterial oxygen.

18. What is a code?

The word *code* is used in hospitals to refer to a patient who is in cardiopulmonary arrest. When a code occurs, the code team is paged to rush to the patient's side to begin immediate resuscitation efforts. All residents in the hospital are trained in advanced cardiac life support (ACLS). The first senior resident to arrive at the patient's side should take on the role of the team leader, according to standard ACLS protocol. In a code, resuscitation first involves securing the ABCs: airway, breathing, and circulation. If a patient is not breathing, intubation may be necessary. An anesthesia team can be called to help with airway management if necessary. Chest compressions are used if the patient is pulseless.

If a patient is found to be in ventricular fibrillation or pulseless ventricular tachycardia, early defibrillation is necessary. If the patient's heart rhythm does not return to normal sinus rhythm (NSR) after receiving a shock, epinephrine is administered with alternating shocks in hopes of restoring NSR. Other medications according to the ACLS algorithm may be used, depending on the underlying rhythms of the patient.

19. What happens if a patient has electrical activity on the heart monitor, but does not have a pulse?

This is referred to as pulseless electrical activity (PEA), which is not a shockable rhythm. In this case, the code team has to determine the etiology of the PEA and try to reverse the underlying cause. A mnemonic known as the 5 H's and 5 T's is commonly used to determine the cause. These criteria are listed in Table 9-3. While the team is trying to find the underlying cause, it is important to continue CPR. Epinephrine may be administered every 3 to 5 minutes.

TABLE 9-3. POSSIBLE CAUSES OF PULSELESS ELECTRICAL ACTIVITY

5 H's	5 T's
Hypovolemia	Tablets or toxins (drug overdose)
Hypoxia	Tamponade (cardiac)
Hydrogen ions (acidosis)	Tension pneumothorax
Hypothermia	Thrombosis (myocardial infarction)
Hyperkalemia	Thrombosis (pulmonary embolism)

20. What happens if a patient does not have any activity on the heart monitor?

This is referred to as asystole. If a patient is in asystole, defibrillation does not help. However, in rare cases, the patient is actually in "fine" ventricular fibrillation (which may appear to be asystole), and some physicians will try defibrillation. Occasionally transcutaneous pacing, electrical pacing of the heart through the patient's chest wall, is used to try to regain a heart rhythm. It is important to continue CPR in this scenario, and just as in PEA, epinephrine may be given every 3 to 5 minutes.

21. How can a medical student help in a code?

Medical students can be very helpful in a code. Chest compressions are tiring and thus require a rotation of several people. Medical students can definitely be involved in this rotation. It is important to note that providing appropriate chest compressions is critical in trying to maintain circulation to vital organs (i.e., the brain). It is also helpful for students to look through medical records to provide the code team with the patient's diagnosis, any relevant medical history, and recent laboratory values. Finally, all patients in a code will have a blood draw to check arterial blood gas (ABG). Medical students are often allowed to draw the blood and can run the sample to the laboratory for immediate reading. Medical students should always carry materials for an ABG with them and know where the laboratory is located.

22. If a patient is physically unable or not mentally competent to make decisions, who makes medical decisions for the patient?

In this situation, physicians must determine whether the patient has created an advanced directive. An advanced directive is a document in which a patient states his or her wishes about future medical care in the event that he or she becomes unable to communicate or make competent decisions. A durable power of attorney and a living will are types of advanced directives. A durable power of attorney means that the patient has designated someone to make decisions for him or her if he or she is unable to do so. A living will is a document in which a patient has documented the forms of medical care he or she wishes to receive.

23. Who makes decisions for the patient if he or she does not have an advanced directive?

In this case, the patient's family can be consulted to make medical decisions. If the patient's condition requires emergency intervention and no family or advanced directive is available, the physician may make decisions that are best for the patient's medical care.

24. Where can patients receive care once they have been stabilized and no longer require ICU care?

When physicians feel a patient has stabilized but needs more time to recover, the patient can be deemed "floor status" and moved to the general floor. The ICU is a difficult place for patients to rest because of the distractions of extra machines and monitoring devices in the ICU. In addition, a 1-day stay in the ICU is much more expensive than a stay on the general floor. As the number of beds in the ICU is limited, it is also necessary to move patients to the floor so that the ICU team can care for other, more critically ill patients.

KEY POINTS: INTENSIVE CARE UNIT 

1. The ICU is a specialized area of the hospital designated for patients who are critically ill and may require increased monitoring, hemodynamic support, or airway support.
2. The ICU typically has a higher provider-to-patient ratio than an inpatient floor.
3. An ICU patient's management plan is typically recorded and presented in a system-based format because these patients' conditions are far more complex.
4. An advanced directive is a document in which a patient states his or her wishes about future medical care in the event that he or she becomes unable to communicate or make competent decisions. If the patient does not have an advanced directive, the family should be consulted. If the family is unavailable, the physician must make decisions in the best interest of the patient's medical care.

CHAPTER 10

THE DISCHARGE PROCESS

Mitesh S. Patel

1. **Who makes the decision that a patient can be discharged?**
Although residents, medical students, and other staff can anticipate a patient's discharge, the attending physician makes the final decision regarding the appropriate time for patient discharge.

2. **When is a patient determined to be appropriate for discharge?**
The decision to discharge a patient from the hospital depends on resolving or stabilizing the acute medical issues that the patient originally presented with and the issues that may not be manageable in the outpatient setting. In addition, proper follow-up of laboratory results and diagnostic tests, as well as determination of transportation and destination upon leaving the hospital, will need to be arranged.

3. **List the common steps involved in the discharge paperwork.**
The paperwork involved in the discharge process varies across institutions. A list of the common components of a typical set of discharge paperwork is displayed in Table 10-1.

TABLE 10-1. COMPONENTS OF THE DISCHARGE PAPERWORK

Patient team information	A listing of the attending, residents, medical students, and other staff who were involved in the patient's care.
Primary care physician	Name and contact information of the patient's primary care physician and any other physicians who are involved in the patient's outpatient care.
Diagnosis	The diagnosis the patient was treated for during this acute hospitalization and any previous medical diagnoses that the patient has been given.
Medications	A list of the medications and dosages prescribed for the patient to take upon discharge from the hospital. It is important to highlight the medication changes that have been made for the patient.
Unresolved issues	Any issues that physicians and staff should pay special attention to during outpatient follow-up visits.
Laboratory results	May include laboratory tests upon admission, any important laboratory results during the hospital stay, and any laboratory data that should be followed in the outpatient setting.
Procedures	A list of procedures performed during the inpatient stay along with any diagnostic results or complications of the procedures.

(Continued)

TABLE 10-1. COMPONENTS OF THE DISCHARGE PAPERWORK (CONTINUED)	
Follow-up	A list of the patient's appointments for follow-up care after discharge from the hospital.
Patient education	Information regarding the patient's hospital stay, medical diagnoses, and management of medical issues in the outpatient setting.
Discharge physical examination	A report of the pertinent positive and negative aspects from the physical examination on the day of discharge.
Clinical course	A summary of the patient's clinical course during the inpatient stay, including a summary of the reasons for hospital admission, important events that occurred, and medical management during the admission.

4. **What should be included in the discharge physical examination?**
Almost all hospitals require that a patient have a physical examination conducted by a physician on the day of discharge. A complete physical examination should be performed, with special attention being paid to any portions of the examination that are related to the patient's reason for hospital admission. For example, if a patient was admitted for mental status changes, a Mini Mental State Examination and a full neurologic assessment should be performed. Other important items to include in the discharge examination are the patient's weight and vital signs.

5. **What are the possible locations that a patient can be discharged to?**
The majority of patients will be discharged to go home. However, some patients may require additional medical attention that cannot be provided at home. The patient can either go home and have a visiting nurse provide some aspects of home medical care or he or she may go to another facility (such as an extended care facility) for further care. Common locations after discharge besides home include a subacute care facility, skilled nursing facility, rehabilitation center, nursing home, hospice, and long-term care hospital.

6. **Describe the role of a discharge coordinator.**
The discharge process can become very complex with the large number of tasks that must be accomplished before completion of patient discharge. In fact, many larger institutions are now hiring a permanent staff member, referred to as the discharge coordinator, discharge planner, or discharge nurse, to facilitate many of the tasks needed to arrange for a patient to have a smooth transition out of the hospital. These may include arranging for ambulance pick-up, visiting nurses, durable medical equipment, and family assistance in determining an ideal extended care facility.

7. **What is a discharge order?**
The discharge order is the official order within the patient's chart indicating that all other tasks have been completed, and the patient is ready to be discharged from the hospital. The order is commonly written in the same location (the patient's written or electronic chart) as orders for medications and diagnostic tests. The order must include the location to which the patient is being discharged, such as home or another service. Some hospitals also require writing who the patient is being discharged with, such as father, daughter, or spouse. A typical order might be written as "Discharge patient home with spouse."

8. **How does a discharge affect the flow of patients through the hospital?**
Each hospital has a maximum number of beds available. Once these beds are filled, no more patients can be moved to the inpatient floors for admission. The patients requiring medical care often face increased waiting times or may have to obtain care in the emergency department (ED) for an extended period. Sometimes hospitals will even tell ambulances to take patients to an alternate hospital if possible (called a *diversion*). Once a patient is discharged, a number of events are set off as displayed in Figure 10-1. Each discharge opens a bed for another patient who needs to be admitted. Once the newly admitted patient is transferred to the bed, a space opens up wherever that patient was, usually in the ED. This allows another patient to move from the ED waiting room into the ED to receive medical attention.

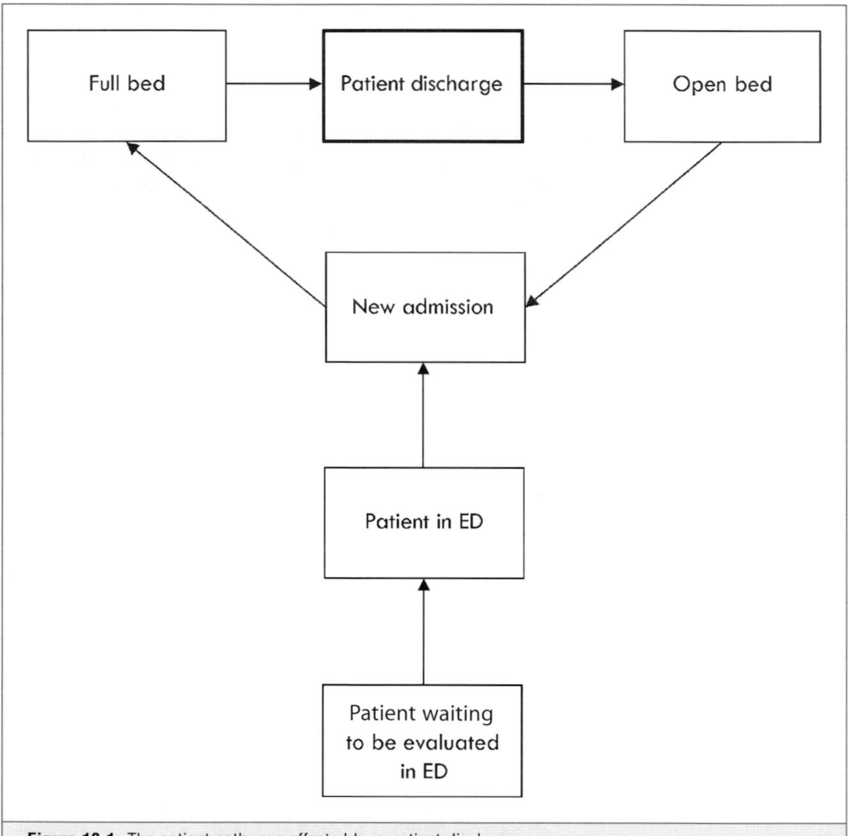

Figure 10-1. The patient pathways affected by a patient discharge.

9. **What is included within the patient discharge instructions?**
Patient education, medications/prescriptions, and follow-up medical care visits are the main components of the discharge instructions. The patient education portion should include a discussion of the patient's medical issues and any appropriate instructions for caution and care once out of the hospital. For example, patients with eye surgery may be told to take caution in avoiding eye contact when washing their face with soap and to

take care by wearing sunglasses while outside or in bright lights. The medications portion should include an updated list of the patient's medication regimen upon being discharged. The patient should be told specifically about any new medications or changes to their old medication regimen. A list of the patient's future medical care visits should be provided to ensure appropriate follow-up care and to inform the patient of any newly made appointments. Sometimes follow-up visits are required but could not be made while the patient was in the hospital. The patient should be told specifically about these visits and advised on how to schedule an appointment.

10. **How are follow-up appointments scheduled when a patient is discharged?**
There are several people in charge of setting up a patient's follow-up appointments, and there are several ways of scheduling the appointment. Larger hospitals have discharge coordinators who are in charge of calling physician offices and scheduling the patient's appointments. At other hospitals and even in many of the larger hospitals, residents and medical students will be responsible for calling another facility to schedule an appointment. Some patients may have very inflexible schedules, and in this case it may be easiest to give the patient instructions on how to schedule their own appointments. However, with this method, no one is checking to confirm that the patient actually makes the appointment, and this can cause problems in the future. The various ways to schedule an appointment vary by institution but involve calling the physician's office, scheduling an appointment online, or having the physician's office call the patient at a later date to schedule the appointment.

11. **Why are many patients evaluated by a physical therapist before discharge?**
A physical therapist is an excellent resource for determining whether a patient will be safe at home. Physical therapists are experts in evaluating whether or not a patient can safely walk around their house, transfer from bed to a chair, or get to the bathroom. In addition, they can help provide extra resources, such as walkers for patients with balance difficulty.

12. **List the most common reasons for delays in the discharge process.**
The most common reason a patient remains in the hospital rather than being discharged is an unresolved medical issue. However, because this is usually the reason for their admission, it is not typically considered a delay unless it is due to unusual circumstances. Some of the more common reasons for delays include pending laboratory tests and diagnostic tests, transportation issues, and waiting for beds to become available in extended care facilities. Patients who have laboratory values that are tracked during their course of stay may need a final set of laboratory tests on the day of discharge. It is important to have their blood drawn early in the morning so that results can come back promptly. Many physicians will even write the order for the blood draw during the night before discharge. Patients in the hospital usually do not have their car or vehicle of transportation with them. Therefore, it is important to let the patient know ahead of time that a family member or friend should plan on picking them up from the hospital. Out-of-hospital care facilities such as rehabilitation centers may often be full. Therefore, it is not uncommon for patients to remain in the hospital a few extra days until a spot becomes available for them.

KEY POINTS: THE DISCHARGE PROCESS

1. The decision to discharge a patient from the hospital depends on resolving or stabilizing the acute medical issues that the patient originally presented with and the issues that may not be manageable in the outpatient setting.
2. Almost all hospitals require that a patient must have a physical examination conducted by a physician on the day of discharge.
3. Many larger institutions are now hiring a permanent staff member, referred to as the discharge coordinator, discharge planner, or discharge nurse, to facilitate many of the tasks needed to arrange for a patient to have a smooth transition out of the hospital.
4. Patient education, medications/prescriptions, and follow-up medical care visits are the main components of discharge instructions.

OUTPATIENT MEDICINE

Nitin K. Gupta

CHAPTER 11

1. **What is outpatient medicine?**
   Outpatient medicine (or ambulatory medicine) refers to medical care that is delivered without admission to the hospital. The patient enters the facility where care is provided and then leaves once care is delivered.

2. **What types of patients should not receive outpatient care?**
   Outpatient care is NOT appropriate if the patient is unstable and requires close monitoring or if subsequent treatment for the patient cannot be delivered at home (e.g., intravenous [IV] fluid or medications).

3. **Where is outpatient care delivered?**
   Outpatient medical care is delivered in a number of settings. The most common site is the outpatient clinic (e.g., a doctor's office). There are several types of outpatient clinics including primary care clinics, specialty clinics, and urgent/emergency care clinics. Outpatient care can also be delivered in surgical sites and procedural offices/suites.

4. **What is primary care?**
   Primary care is the act of a healthcare provider that serves as the initial assessment of care for a patient. Primary care clinics are conducted in the outpatient setting and involve family physicians, internal medicine physicians, pediatricians, and some obstetrics/gynecology physicians.

5. **Who should receive care at a primary care clinic?**
   All individuals should establish care in a primary care clinic. If possible, the clinic should be conveniently located and easily accessible.

6. **Why do patients come to a primary care clinic?**
   Most new medical complaints are first evaluated at a primary care clinic. The complaint may be addressed within that clinic or the patient may be referred to a specialized clinic. However, if the patient is having severe symptoms that suggest an acute life-threatening process, the patient should present to the nearest emergency department.

   Patients with previously presented complaints or chronic diseases may receive follow-up care in a primary care clinic if the healthcare provider at that clinic is comfortable managing the patient's illness. For example, a diabetic patient may visit a primary care physician every 3 to 6 months to assess hemoglobin A1c and glucose levels.

   Patients who originally presented to the emergency department or were recently admitted to the hospital usually follow up in a primary care clinic once their more immediate concerns are addressed and they have been discharged from the hospital. For example, an 85-year-old man admitted to the hospital with lobar pneumonia would be seen by his primary care provider after discharge from the hospital to ensure proper recovery.

   A patient may also receive heath maintenance examinations at a primary care clinic. For example, a healthy teenager may present to the primary care clinic for a physical examination required for participation in athletics.

7. **List the types of healthcare providers who deliver care in a primary care clinic.** A list of primary care providers along with their required training and medical roles is displayed in Table 11-1.

TABLE 11-1. TYPES OF PRIMARY CARE PROVIDERS

Health Care Provider	Training and Medical Role
Internists	These are physicians who have completed a 3-year residency in internal medicine. These physicians will take care of the general health care needs of adults.
Pediatricians	These are physicians who have completed a 3-year residency in pediatrics. These physicians will mostly care for individuals younger than age 18.
Gynecologists	These are physicians who have completed a residency training program in obstetrics and gynecology (3 to 4 years). These physicians provide routine gynecologic care (Pap smears, breast examinations, birth control care, etc.). They also play the role of a medical specialist and see patients referred by nongynecologic physicians for gynecologic concerns.
Family physicians	These are physicians who have completed a 3-year residency in family medicine. They may take care of adults and/or children. They may also provide gynecologic and/or obstetric care.
Geriatricians	These are physicians who have completed a 3-year residency in either internal medicine or family medicine and have received additional training in caring for older patients with multiple medical problems (often a fellowship in geriatrics). They serve the general health needs of adults who are usually older than age 65 and often have several complicated medical issues.
Med/Peds	These are physicians who have completed a 4-year combined residency in both internal medicine and pediatrics. They care for patients of all ages but generally do not provide gynecologic care. These physicians often care for children with chronic diseases and can remain the primary care provider as the patient becomes an adult.
Nurse practitioners and physician assistants	These are individuals who may provide general health care for a variety of patients. They are not licensed physicians and usually provide care under the supervision of an appropriate physician.

8. **List the staff seen within an outpatient clinic along with their roles.** The various staff within an outpatient clinic are displayed in Table 11-2 along with their training and role within the clinic.

TABLE 11-2. MEDICAL STAFF WITHIN A HEALTH CARE CLINIC

Medical Staff	Training and Medical Role
Attending physician	A physician who has completed medical school and residency. The attending is ultimately responsible for the care provided to the patient and must agree with the final assessment and plan.

(Continued)

TABLE 11-2. MEDICAL STAFF WITHIN A HEALTH CARE CLINIC (CONTINUED)

Medical Staff	Training and Medical Role
Resident physician	A physician who has completed medical school and is currently in a residency program. In most outpatient clinics affiliated with an academic institution, the resident is the initial physician who speaks with and examines a patient, performs a physical examination, and comes up with a preliminary plan. He or she then staffs with the supervising attending.
Nurse	There may be a variety of types of nurses with different education training among the various outpatient clinics. A nurse is likely to be the one in charge of tasks such as administering shots, giving intravenous medications, or drawing blood. The nurse in some clinics also does the work of a medical assistant.
Medical assistant (MA)	The medical assistant is typically a staff member who transfers the patient into the examination room, obtains and records the vital signs, asks about the chief complaint, and then cleans the room after the patient leaves so that it is ready for the next patient.

9. **Describe a typical day in an outpatient clinic.**
A typical schedule in an outpatient clinic begins between 7 and 9 AM. Daily responsibilities include patient evaluations, which are scheduled back-to-back, and note keeping. In clinics with electronic charts, notes are usually dictated and typed by an outside source. Once typed, they are available to the attending physician to proofread and sign and then become a part of the electronic records. However, in other clinics, notes are hand-written into paper charts. A typical full day ends between 4 and 6 PM.
It is not uncommon for physicians to work half-days, such as 8 AM to 12 noon or 1 to 5 PM.

10. **How long are patient visits within the outpatient setting?**
The length of a patient visit depends on the reason for the evaluation. Yearly health maintenance examinations are usually scheduled for 45 minutes to 1 hour. Return visits for a chronic condition, such as diabetes, are usually scheduled for 15 minutes. New patient consultations at specialty clinics are usually scheduled for 30 or 60 minutes depending on the clinic.

11. **What is a medical student's role in the outpatient clinic?**
In most clinics, after the patient has been transferred to the clinic room, the medical student will first see the patient alone. The student should introduce himself or herself as a medical student working with the patient's physician, and then inform the patient that the attending will later be in to see the patient as well. The medical student should gather the history and conduct a physical examination. The student will then present the pertinent history and physical examination findings to the attending physician. Most attendings will also expect the student to provide an assessment and plan.

12. **Describe the evaluation of a new patient with a new complaint.**
A new patient encounter should begin by obtaining a full history and performing a full physical examination. Key elements of the history include history of present illness, past medical history, family history, social history, current medications and dosages, and drug allergies. A full physical examination should be performed to establish a baseline examination for future visits and future complaints. These visits are typically scheduled for 45 minutes to 1 hour.

13. Describe the evaluation of an established patient with a new complaint.
Although it is important to obtain a thorough history, it should be focused around the patient's new complaint and previous medical conditions. A focused physical examination should be performed to further assess the differential diagnosis that was formed while the history was taken. These visits are commonly scheduled for a little as 15 minutes.

14. Describe the evaluation of a patient returning for follow-up care of a previous complaint.
Before seeing a patient for a return visit regarding a chronic condition, the student should read the most recent follow-up note and in particular the plan stated at the end. Then the student can ask the patient if the plan was followed. The visit should focus on new developments since the most recent visit. These include control of symptoms, any interim exacerbations of the condition or related hospital visits, any changes in medications, medication compliance, and any relevant changes in social or family history. A focused physical examination should be performed. If laboratory tests or studies are generally used to assess the patient's progress, the student should check the patient's record for the results. If they are not in the chart, ask if they have been performed. If the laboratory results have not been obtained, include this information in the patient's plan when presenting the patient to the physician.

15. What is a health maintenance examination (HME)?
An HME is typically conducted annually and involves an overall assessment of a patient's health history, medical risk factors, physical examination, and required laboratory or diagnostic testing. Appropriate patient education is also provided to encourage patients to be aware of their health status and methods for improvement.

16. Describe the evaluation of a patient presenting for a regular check-up (HME).
For an HME, a complete history and physical examination should be conducted. In this case, having the patient's previous medical record is helpful so that while in the patient's room, the student can simply review and confirm the previous data. If this information is not available, the student should ask about the patient's past medical history, medications, and allergies, and then ask if there have been any changes to other parts of the history. A complete history of present illness should be obtained if the patient has a new complaint at the time of the HME. For female patients, reproductive/gynecologic issues should be addressed including description of menstrual cycles, number of gestations, number of live-birth pregnancies, number of abortions, most recent Pap smear, and any previous abnormal Pap smear results. A complete review of systems should be obtained. The student should also determine whether the patient is up to date with his or her vaccines and age-appropriate screening studies. In addition, patients should be asked about general safety practices, such as seatbelt usage and sunscreen protection. These visits are typically scheduled for 45 minutes to 1 hour.

17. Describe the way in which a patient presenting for follow-up from an emergency department or hospital discharge should be addressed in the setting of a primary care clinic.
The medical record from the hospital should be reviewed, including the discharge summary if available. Note the symptoms with which the patient presented at admission, the clinical course, discharge medications, the discharge diagnosis, and whether any issues were unresolved. Focus the medical history on current symptoms and medication compliance. Check the discharge instructions to determine whether any follow-up care such as suture removal is required.

18. What is a specialty clinic?
This clinic is for patients whose problems require the expertise of a specialist in a specific area of medicine such as cardiology or rheumatology.

19. Describe the pathways in which patients might arrive at a specialty clinic.
Patients can be referred to a specialty clinic through several pathways, including from a primary care physician, from the emergency department, after discharge from the hospital, and from another specialty clinic.

20. Provide examples of specialty clinics.
Specialty clinics tend to follow the organ systems. A list of common clinics is provided in Table 11-3.

TABLE 11-3. COMMON SPECIALTY CLINICS
Hematology/oncology
Gastroenterology
Cardiology
Nephrology
Rheumatology
Pulmonology
Infectious diseases
Allergy
Endocrinology
Dermatology
Neurology
Ophthalmology
Surgery
Urology

21. What information should be gathered when a new patient presents in a specialty clinic?
If the patient is at a specialty clinic for a new patient visit, perform a complete history, paying specific attention to the symptoms that caused the primary physician to refer the patient. Many subspecialty clinics perform a focused physical examination with a complete examination of pertinent organ systems (e.g., a complete abdominal examination in a gastroenterology clinic or a complete neurologic examination in a neurology clinic). Be sure to look at the patient's previous medical record and notes from referring physicians. Determine the reason for the referral, what diagnostic work-up has already been completed, and what treatment options have been attempted, along with their associated success or failure rates.

22. What information should be gathered during a return visit in a specialty clinic?
During a return visit, the student should obtain a focused history and physical examination. Ask the patient about changes in symptoms since the previous visit as well as about side effects from new medications prescribed at the last visit. Look at the plan from the previous visit to determine if it has been followed. Find out whether the patient had any problems following the plan. Most importantly, find out whether the plan resulted in any improvement or even worsening in the patient's medical condition.

23. How should a medical student conduct a patient presentation in an outpatient clinic?

Student presentations should be as efficient as possible because there is not much time between patients in the outpatient setting. Remember, attendings still have to see the patient after you! Start with the patient's name, age, sex, and reason for visit (chief complaint, reason for referral, or follow up). Give a concise history of the presenting illness (be complete if it is a new patient; only mention pertinent or new information for established patients). Present pertinent information from the other parts of the history. For physical examination, structure the presentation based on attending preference. Most outpatient attendings only want pertinent positive and negative aspects, but some may want additional information. Then provide a brief assessment and offer a plan if possible.

24. List the various methods of documentation for a patient visit.

Although more and more clinics are beginning to use an online system for patient documentation, many clinics still use handwritten documentation. The common methods of documentation are described in Table 11-4.

TABLE 11-4. METHODS OF DOCUMENTATION

Write by hand	The visit is documented in a paper chart by someone handwriting the note.
Type on computer	The visit is documented in an electronic record system by someone typing up the note and submitting it to the record system.
Dictation	The visit is documented in an electronic record system by someone dictating the note over the phone (or onto a cassette tape) to an outside service. The outside service types up the notes and then sends them back for the physician to edit and submit to the record system.

25. Describe the dictation process.

In many outpatient clinics, documentation of patient visits is in the form of electronic medical records. In these clinics, it is common for notes to be dictated over the phone to an outside service, which then types the notes and sends them back to the physician to edit and submit to the record system. A common technique for beginning a dictation proceeds in the following order:

1. Name of the person dictating
2. Name of the physician the patient saw
3. The patient's name (it often helps to spell the patient's name)
4. Patient identification number
5. Patient's date of birth
6. Date of the visit
7. The type of clinic the patient was seen in

For example, a medical student could say "This is medical student John Smith dictating a note for Dr. Jones. Patient name is Robert Ray, patient number 34567890, date of birth February 4th, 1982, seen on May 8, 2006, in the outpatient cardiology clinic."

The main portion of the dictated note should contain all key elements of the visit including the following: chief complaint, history of present illness, (past medical, social, and family histories if they relate to the present visit), a list of current medications, a list of drug allergies, a physical examination, and an assessment and plan.

Although a dictated note is similar to a handwritten note in format, there are some important features to keep in mind when dictating a note. All grammar must be explicitly stated; otherwise, it is up to the discretion of the person typing the note. For example, if you are listing past medical history it might be appropriate to say, "Past medical history, colon, next line, number 1, asthma, next line, number 2, coronary artery disease, next line, number 3, diabetes mellitus." It is also helpful to spell out words that might be difficult to spell such as the names of medications, certain diseases, etc. Also, whenever starting a new paragraph, say "new paragraph." At the end of the dictation, state that the dictation is over. For example, "this ends the dictation on patient Robert Ray."

Initially, it may be difficult to dictate a note properly. Outlining the note on paper before dictation can help to establish a routine of speaking for future use. Over time, the dictation process will become much easier.

26. Explain the process of providing a prescription.
A prescription can either be handwritten on a paper pad or be printed out from a computer. All prescriptions, however, should include the name of the patient, the date, the name of the medication, dispensing information, patient instructions, number of refills, the name of the physician, and a signature of the physician (his or her DEA number is also required for certain drugs). The name of the medication can either be written as a brand name or as a generic version. If it is not otherwise specified, a pharmacy may substitute a generic for a brand name medication. If a physician wants the exact medication to be given, he or she should write on the prescription "dispensed as written" or "DAW." The dispensing instructions include the dosage of the medication, the size of the pills, route of delivery, frequency, and the number of refills. Patient instructions should explain to the patient how to take the medication in a manner that is easily understood. Figure 11-1 displays a sample prescription with a brief description of each component.

27. When should the patient return for another visit?
The length of time before a patient should return for another visit depends on the reason the patient presented and the discretion of the physician. After an HME, a patient does not need to return until the following year, unless another concern arises. For a condition such as strep throat, a patient is usually not asked to return unless the condition does not improve or symptoms worsen. For most chronic conditions, a patient is expected to return to the clinic for follow-up at regularly scheduled intervals on the basis of the physician's preference. For example, patients with diabetes mellitus are usually seen every 3 to 6 months for follow-up.

28. Describe the time constraints in an outpatient clinic.
Outpatient clinics are designed to offer care to the maximum number of patients as is possible. Clinics often schedule patients back-to-back and may double-book patients when extra help (medical students, residents, or physician assistants) is available. The medical student should try to see patients quickly, present efficiently, and gather necessary paperwork (i.e., consult forms, prescriptions, and patient education handouts) while waiting to staff a patient with the attending. Also, spend time gathering information efficiently. Some information is more easily gathered from old notes, other information is best taken directly from patients, and other information might best be found in medical reference books.

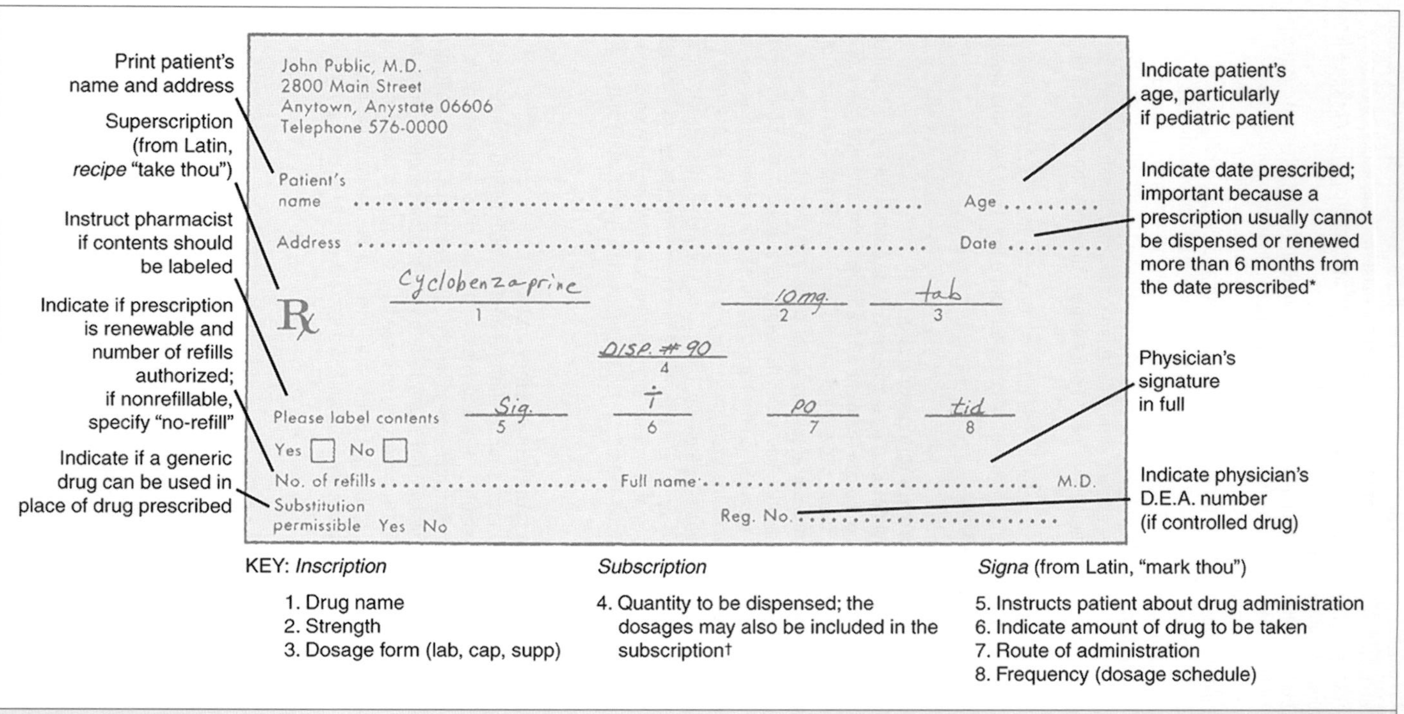

Figure 11-1. A sample prescription with a description of each component. (From Ferri FF: Practical Guide to the Care of the Medical Patient, ed 7, Philadelphia, Mosby, 2007, with permission.)

KEY POINTS: OUTPATIENT MEDICINE 

1. Outpatient care is not appropriate if the patient is unstable and requires close monitoring or if subsequent treatment for the patient cannot be delivered at home.
2. Primary care is the action of a healthcare provider that serves as the initial assessment of care for a patient. Primary care clinics are conducted in the outpatient setting and involve family physicians, internal medicine physicians, pediatricians, and some obstetrics/gynecology physicians.
3. A health maintenance examination is typically conducted annually and involves an overall assessment of a patient's health history, medical risk factors, physical examination, and required laboratory or diagnostic testing.
4. If a patient is presenting in the outpatient clinic after recent discharge from the emergency department or hospital, it is important to review the discharge summary. Pay special attention to the reasons for the hospital visit, clinical course, discharge diagnosis, changes in medications, and existence of any unresolved issues.
5. Students should be as efficient as possible when presenting patients to staff in the outpatient setting because time is limited and there are usually many patients scheduled in the clinic within 1 day.
6. The methods of medical documentation in the outpatient setting include handwritten notes, typed electronic notes, and verbal dictation.
7. All prescriptions should include the name of the patient, the date, the name of the medication, dispensing information, patient instructions, number of refills, the name of the physician, and a signature of the physician (also his or her DEA number for certain drugs).

CHAPTER 12

PROCEDURES

Derek K. Juang

ESSENTIAL PROCEDURES

Medical students will be expected to be able to perform the following procedures. Follow all standard barrier precautions. Note that in most instances, these procedures should only be performed under supervision. Although steps to perform procedures are provided, by no means should students perform a procedure without requesting permission from a supervising physician.

1. List the usage, materials, and procedural steps of an intravenous (IV) catheter insertion.

Use

For access to administer fluids, blood, or medication.

Materials

IV cannula (angiocatheter or intracatheter), tourniquet, alcohol swab, dressing (Tegaderm), tape.

Steps

1. Choose distal veins on the upper, nondominant extremity first. However, any peripheral vein, the external jugular vein, or even scalp veins may be used.
2. Place the tourniquet proximal to the access site. To help visualize the veins, it may help to lightly tap a finger over the veins. This can cause the vein to bulge slightly.
3. Clean the site with an alcohol swab.
4. Stabilize the vein with your free hand, being sure not to contaminate the sterilized area as displayed in Figure 12-1. This can be done by providing steady traction distal to the puncture site.
5. Enter the vein at about a 20-degree angle. When a "flash" of blood is seen, decrease the angle a bit further and advance 2 mm more to ensure that the needle and the tip of the catheter are in the vein as displayed in Figure 12-2.
6. Advance the IV catheter, and then remove the needle.
7. Secure the IV catheter with dressing and tape.

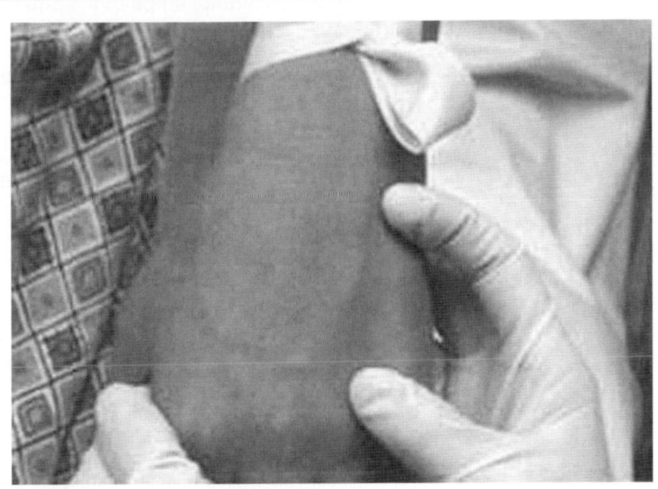

Figure 12-1. Stabilizing the vein during an intravenous catheter insertion. (From Roberts JR, Hedges JR: Clinical Procedures in Emergency Medicine, ed 4, Philadelphia, WB Saunders, 2004, with permission.)

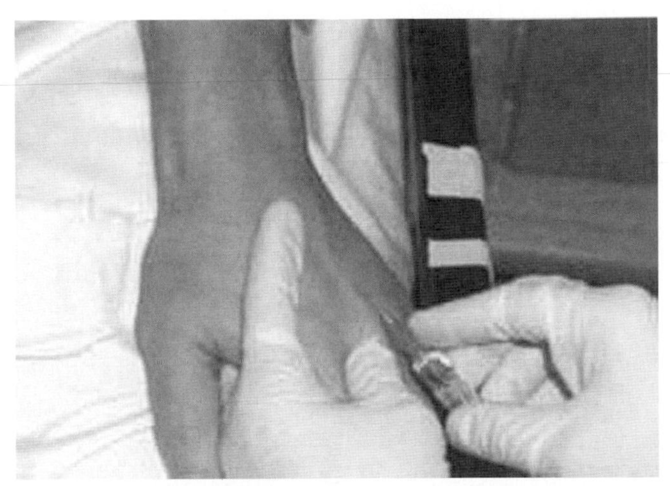

Figure 12-2. Insertion of the needle and catheter into the vein during an intravenous catheter insertion. (From Roberts JR, Hedges JR: Clinical Procedures in Emergency Medicine, ed 4, Philadelphia, WB Saunders, 2004, with permission.)

2. List the usage, necessary materials, and procedural steps of a blood draw for an arterial blood gas (ABG) measurement.

Use

For blood gas determination and analysis.

Materials

Heparinized syringe (a special syringe used for blood gases), 22- to 25-gauge needle (it may be easier to use a butterfly needle), alcohol swab.

Steps

1. The radial artery is used most frequently, and this approach is described here. Verify patency of the collateral circulation with the Allen test. Have the patient make a tight fist. Occlude both the radial and ulnar arteries at the wrist. Have the patient pump his or her fist until the hand is pale. While maintaining pressure on the radial artery, release the ulnar artery. Color should return to the hand within 10 seconds. If the result of this test is positive (color does not return), the radial artery should not be used.
2. It may help to have an assistant hyperextend the patient's wrist and hold the patient's hand in place.
3. Prepare the puncture site with an alcohol swab.
4. Enter the artery with the bevel up at a 60- to 90-degree angle as displayed in Figure 12-3.
5. When a "flash" of blood is seen, slowly withdraw blood. For a blood gas measurement, only 2 to 3 mL are typically needed.
6. Withdraw the needle quickly and apply firm pressure directly over the puncture site.
7. Place the collection tube on ice before taking the sample to the laboratory if required by the hospital.

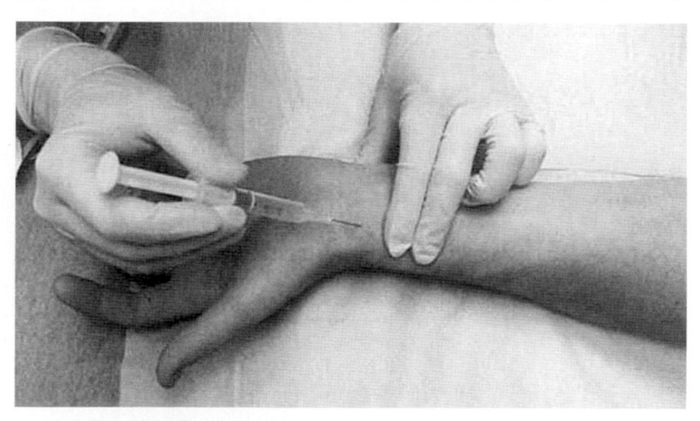

Figure 12-3. Insertion of the needle into the radial artery at a 60- to 90-degree angle during an arterial blood gas. (From Roberts JR, Hedges JR: Clinical Procedures in Emergency Medicine, ed 4, Philadelphia, WB Saunders, 2004, with permission.)

3. List the usage, necessary materials, and procedural steps of an arterial line placement.

Use
For frequent sampling of arterial blood and hemodynamic monitoring when continuous blood pressure readings are necessary.

Materials
20-gauge (or smaller) angiocatheter, arterial line setup per intensive care unit routine (transducer, tubing, and pressure bag with heparinized saline), armboard, dressing (Tegaderm), lidocaine.

Steps
1. The radial artery is used most frequently, and this approach is described here. Verify patency of the collateral circulation with the Allen test, as described earlier.
2. Place an armboard beneath the arm, with a roll of gauze behind the wrist to hyperextend the wrist. Prepare the wrist with an iodine solution, and drape with sterile towels, exposing only the puncture site.
3. Palpate the radial artery. Inject 1% lidocaine above where the pulse is felt.
4. Using a 30-degree angle with the bevel up, advance the angiocatheter into the artery. Once a "flash" of blood is seen in the hub, advance 1 to 2 mm further so that both the needle and catheter are in the artery. Advance the catheter over the needle into the artery.
5. Manually occlude the artery proximally, remove the needle, and connect pressure tubing.
6. Secure the catheter in place with 3-0 silk suture or with sterile dressing.
7. Adjust the transducer's height until it is level with the patient's left atrium. The line will then need to be calibrated on the basis of the respective institution's method.

4. List the usage, necessary materials, and procedural steps of a nasogastric (NG) tube insertion.

Use
For gastrointestinal decompression, stomach lavage, or feeding patients. Contraindicated in patients with nasal or basilar skull fractures.

Materials
NG tube, lubricant jelly, glass of water, straw, tape

Steps
1. Squirt anesthetic into the nose to numb the area if desired.
2. Approximate the amount of tube needed: measure from the xiphoid process, up to the patient's nose, and around the ear, and then add 6 inches more. An example is displayed in Figure 12-4.
3. Run the tube under warm water or wrap tubing around your finger to make it more pliable at the tip.
4. Lubricate the end of the tube.
5. Place the patient's head in flexion, and insert the tube gently along the floor of the nasal passageway.
6. When the tube is in the back of the patient's throat, ask the patient to drink water through the straw. Continue to pass the tube as the patient drinks water until the estimated point is reached.
7. Secure the tube by taping the tube to the patient's nose or forehead.
8. If the patient can talk without difficulty and gastric fluid returns, the tube should be located in the stomach. Also verify placement by blowing air into the tube and listening for a stomach gurgle with your stethoscope. Obtain an x-ray if unsure and before starting any feedings.

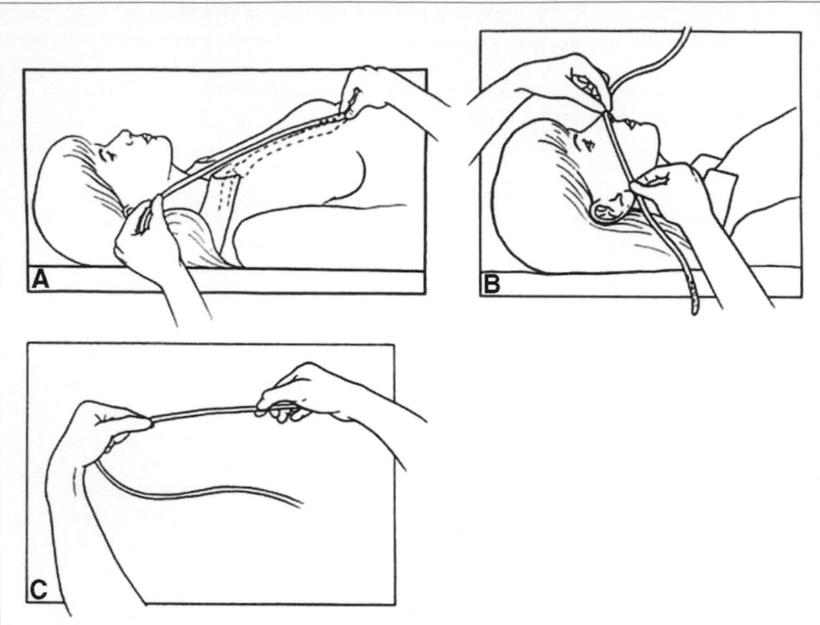

Figure 12-4. A method for approximating the length of tubing necessary during a nasogastric tube insertion. (From Roberts JR, Hedges JR: Clinical Procedures in Emergency Medicine, ed 4, Philadelphia, WB Saunders, 2004, with permission.)

5. **List the usage, necessary materials, and procedural steps of a bladder catheterization.**

Use

For urinary retention, obtaining clean urine samples, and monitoring urine output. Do not perform if blood is seen at urethral meatus, pelvic injury is suspected, a high-riding prostate is present on pelvic examination, or if you are concerned about acute prostatitis.

Materials

Usually come in a prepackaged Foley catheter insertion tray.

Steps

1. Open the package and put on gloves using sterile procedure. Open the iodine preparation solution and soak cotton balls. Apply sterile drapes.
2. Inflate and deflate the balloon on the catheter to ensure proper functioning. Coat the end with sterile lubricant.
3. Use one hand to expose the urethral meatus if necessary (spreading the labia in females or retracting the foreskin in males). This hand is now considered unsterile.
4. Prepare the urethral meatus with iodine solution on cotton balls.

5. Place the catheter into the urethra and advance until urine returns. As soon as urine returns, advance a few more centimeters and then inflate the balloon with saline.
6. If catheter cannot be inserted, try a larger Foley catheter or a coude catheter (has a curved tip).
7. When removing the Foley catheter, remember to first deflate the balloon!

6. List the usage, necessary materials, and procedural steps of a laceration repair.

Use

Most traumatic lacerations that will not stop bleeding on their own will require suture. In addition, suturing a laceration may help the wound heal faster.

Materials

For skin lacerations, use nylon 6-0 for the face, 5-0 for the hands and feet, and 4-0 for the body. For deep lacerations, use Vicryl 5-0 for the face, 4-0 for the hands and feet, and 3-0 for the body. Sterile saline, gauze, lidocaine 1% or LET (a topical anesthetic composed of lidocaine, epinephrine, and tetracaine), suture scissors.

Steps

1. Cleanse the wound with sterile saline and dry with gauze.
2. Inject 1% lidocaine around the wound, or apply LET for >20 minutes. Do not use LET if the laceration is on an extreme distal portion of the body such as a toe or tip of a finger.
3. Using interrupted stitches, close the wound, leaving 3 to 5 mm between each stitch. An example is displayed in Figure 12-5. Because most traumatic lacerations are uneven, it is difficult to use running or subcuticular stitches to close these wounds.
4. May also close linear or scalp lacerations similarly with staples rather than suture if desired.

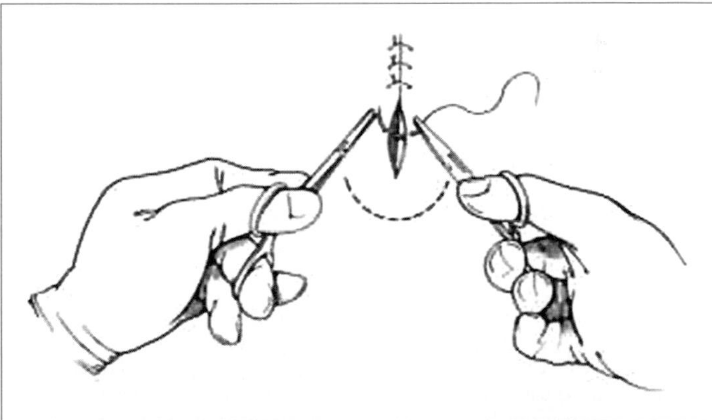

Figure 12-5. Closing a wound using interrupted stitches. (From Roberts JR, Hedges JR: Clinical Procedures in Emergency Medicine, ed 4, Philadelphia, WB Saunders, 2004, with permission.)

7. **List the usage, necessary materials, and procedural steps of an incision and drainage (I&D).**

Use
To drain an abscess.

Materials
Scalpel with no. 11 blade, lidocaine 1%, packing strip, iodine preparation, sterile dressing, gauze, sterile saline.

Steps
1. Prepare the site with iodine.
2. Inject lidocaine and create a wheal over the incision site.
3. When the area is numb, incise directly over the abscess pocket.
4. Express the contents of the abscess by applying pressure with both hands and then cleanse the wound with sterile saline. Be sure to remove as much of the abscess contents as possible. Be careful not to stick your finger within the abscess cavity if the abscess is suspected to be from a patient injecting drugs into his or her subcutaneous space.
5. Pack the open wound with appropriately sized and moistened packing gauze.

ADVANCED PROCEDURES

The following are procedures that medical students will probably be asked to assist with or may be able to perform with close supervision.

8. **List the usage, necessary materials, and procedural steps of a lumbar puncture.**

Use
Diagnosis of central nervous system infections, Guillain-Barré syndrome, intracranial hypo- or hypertension, demyelinating disorders, and subarachnoid hemorrhage. Contraindicated if there is a possibility of an intracranial mass, increased intracranial pressure (papilledema), or focal neurologic findings.

Materials
Most hospitals will have all materials needed in a kit, usually including a 20- to 22- gauge needle with a stylet, a 10-mL syringe, four collecting tubes, sterile drapes, chlorhexidine preparation, and lidocaine. Sterile gloves are also needed.

Steps
1. Place the patient in the lateral decubitus position with the neck, back, knees, and hips maximally flexed.
2. Locate the patient's iliac crests; these correspond to the L4–L5 interspace. Feel for the space between the patient's spine in this area. This will be your puncture site.
3. Put on sterile gloves, and prepare the area with an iodine solution.
4. Anesthetize the puncture site with lidocaine. Anesthetize deeper tissues, aspirating before injecting to ensure that the needle has not entered a subarachnoid space or a vessel.

5. Use a 22- or 20-gauge spinal needle. Insert the needle just caudal to the L4 spinous process, keeping pressure on the hub of the stylet to avoid having it displaced from the needle.
6. Aim for the umbilicus. Advance slowly until a "pop" is felt, indicating passage through the longitudinal ligament.
7. Remove the stylet and check for cerebrospinal fluid (CSF) flow. Never advance without replacing the stylet.
8. Once CSF flow is obtained, attach the stopcock with a manometer to measure opening pressure (normal is 70 to 180 mm H_2O).
9. Acquire specimens in four tubes in a specific order: (1) for cell count and differential, (2) for glucose and protein, (3) for culture and Gram's stain, and (4) for cell count and differential. Blood in the CSF may be due to a traumatic lumbar puncture or subarachnoid hemorrhage (SAH). Xanthochromia (centrifuged CSF with a pigmented supernatant) is a sign of SAH.

9. List the usage, necessary materials, and procedural steps of a central venous catheter (Seldinger technique).

Use

To administer fluids and medications (faster than a peripheral line), transvenous pacemaker placement, hemodynamic monitoring.

Materials

Most hospitals will have all materials needed in a kit, usually including a 16- to 18- gauge needle, guidewire, scalpel, 10-mL syringe, a dilator, sterile towels, chlorhexidine preparation, and lidocaine.

Steps

The approach to the right intrajugular (IJ) vein will be described and is displayed in Figure 12-6. The left IJ, subclavian, medial basilica, and femoral veins may also be used for central lines.

1. Use sterile protection (mask, gown, and gloves).
2. Prepare the site with chlorhexidine, drape with sterile towels, and anesthetize the site.
3. With the patient in the Trendelenburg position, use a small needle with a syringe attached to locate the IJ by entering between the apex of the triangle formed by the two heads of the sternocleidomastoid muscle and the clavicle. The usual depth is approximately 2 to 4 cm. Aspirate as you enter. This portion of the procedure is frequently performed under ultrasound guidance.
4. If necessary, detach the syringe from the needle. Pass the guidewire into the vein through the needle (or syringe and needle).
5. Remove the needle. NEVER let go of the guidewire.
6. Nick the skin adjacent to the guidewire with the scalpel, and then insert the dilator as far as possible.
7. Remove the dilator, and pass the central line catheter into the vein. Once the catheter is in place, the guidewire may be removed.
8. Draw back until you see blood, and then flush the line to ensure that it is patent.
9. Secure the line with a suture, and then apply a sterile dressing.
10. Obtain a chest x-ray to verify the position of the line and to assess for pneumothorax. The tip of the catheter should be above the right atrium.
11. To remove the central line, place the patient in the reverse Trendelenburg position. Ask the patient to hum while removing the line to prevent an air embolism.

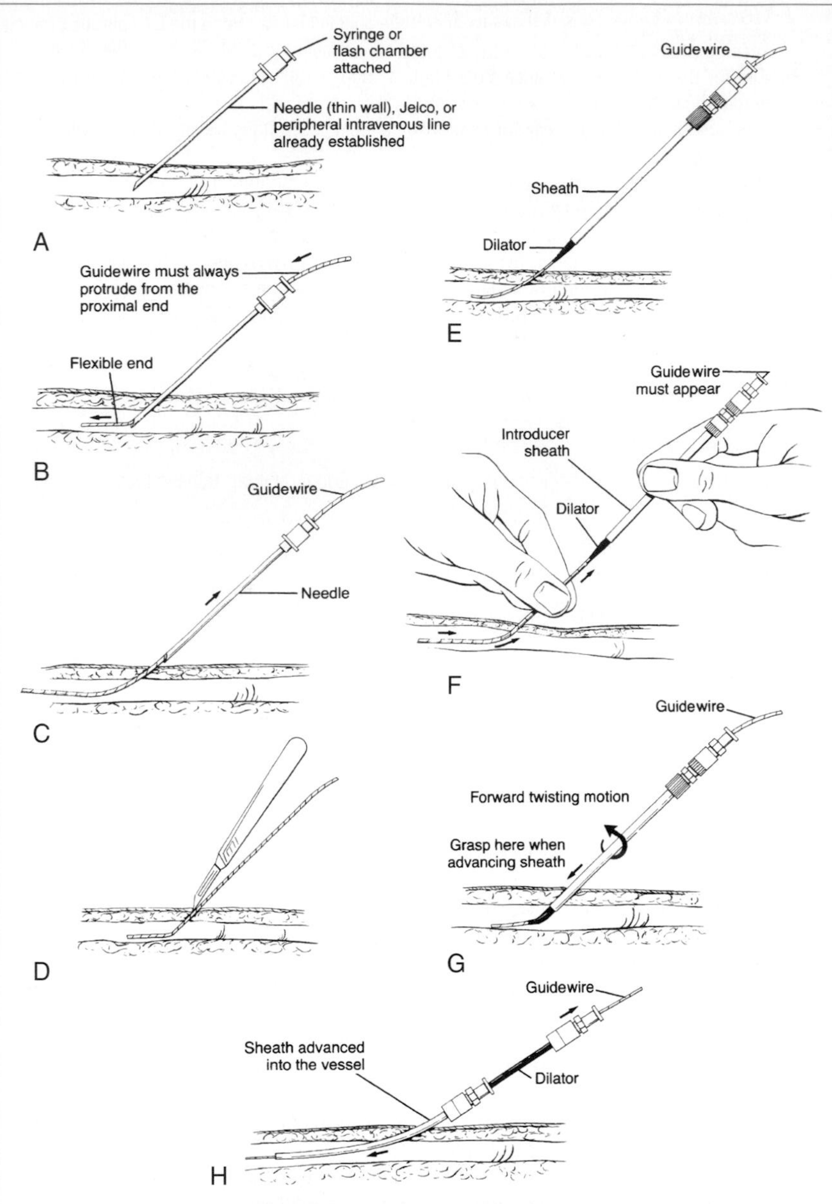

Figure 12-6. An example of the method used to insert a central venous catheter. (From Roberts JR, Hedges JR: Clinical Procedures in Emergency Medicine, ed 4, Philadelphia, WB Saunders, 2004, with permission.)

10. List the usage, necessary materials, and procedural steps of an endotracheal intubation.

Use

Patients who are at risk of losing their airway or need proper respiratory control. Often includes patients in cardiac arrest, patients in respiratory distress, and patients at risk for aspiration.

Materials

Endotracheal tube (ETT), laryngoscope handle and blade, 10-mL syringe, tape, suction equipment.

Steps

1. Use a bag and mask with 100% oxygen to oxygenate the patient for 3 to 5 minutes.
2. Inflate the ETT cuff to ensure patency. Then position the patient in the "sniffing position," with neck flexed and head slightly extended.
3. Use IV sedation unless the patient is nonresponsive. Commonly used sedatives include midazolam, fentanyl, or etomidate.
4. "Scissor" the patient's mouth open by pushing the lower incisors with your thumb and pushing his upper incisors with your index finger.
5. With your left hand, insert the laryngoscope blade into the right side of the patient's mouth, and use the blade to sweep the tongue out of the way. Advance the blade until the epiglottis is seen
6. If using the curved (Macintosh) blade, pass the blade anterior and superior to the epiglottis. If using the straight (Miller) blade, pass the blade posterior and inferior to the epiglottis, occluding it from view.
7. Do not pivot on the patient's maxillary teeth. Instead, raise your arm at a 45-degree angle towards the roof, until you can visualize the vocal cords.
8. While keeping your eyes on the cords, use your right hand to insert the ETT through the cords. In most patients, insert the cord about 21 to 23 cm.
9. Inflate the cuff of the ETT. The tube is probably properly placed if (1) you see condensation in the tube, (2) you hear bilateral, equal breath sounds in the lungs, and no gurgling in the stomach; or (3) end-tidal CO_2 is measured on capnography.
10. Secure the tube with tape.

An example of this procedure is displayed in Figure 12-7.

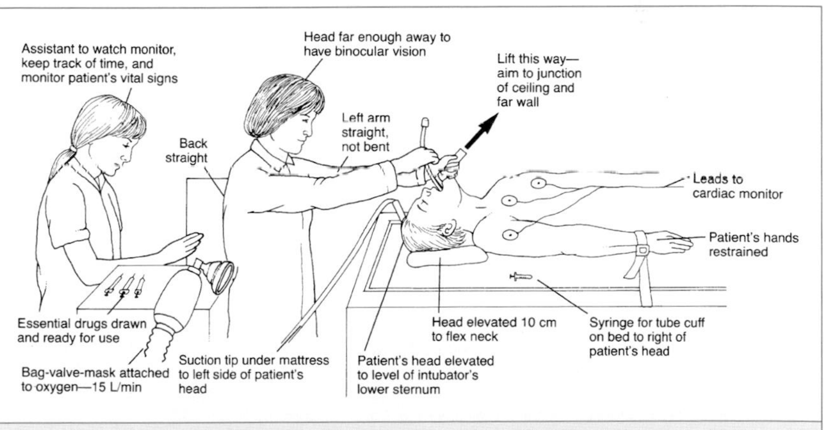

Figure 12-7. Proper positioning for endotracheal intubation. (From Roberts JR, Hedges JR: Clinical Procedures in Emergency Medicine, ed 4, Philadelphia, WB Saunders, 2004, with permission.)

11. List the usage, necessary materials, and procedural steps of a chest tube placement.

Use

To reduce a pneumothorax, drainage of a hemothorax or large pleural effusion.

Materials

Chest tube, Pleur-evac suction unit, tubing, wall suction connection, scalpel, large Kelly clamps (similar to forceps or a hemostat, with a curved end), needle driver, scissors, suture, lidocaine.

Steps

1. Place the patient's ipsilateral arm over his head as displayed in Figure 12-8.
2. Place the puncture site at the mid-axillary line between the fourth and fifth ribs (above the level of the nipple). Anesthetize the area with lidocaine.
3. Make a 2-cm incision parallel to the ribs through the skin, subcutaneous tissues, and intercostal muscles.
4. Bluntly enter the pleural space with a Kelly clamp. Once you enter the pleural space, spread the Kelly clamp to widen the hole in the chest wall.

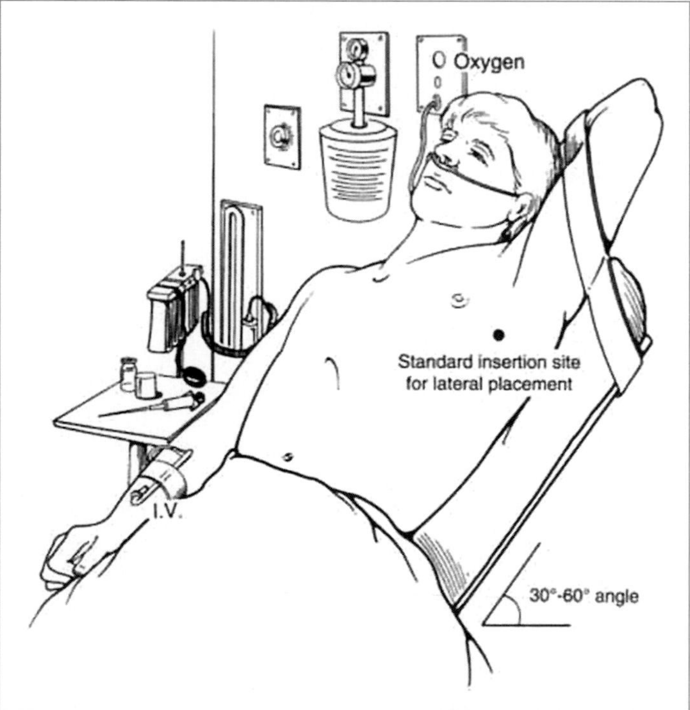

Figure 12-8. Proper positioning for chest tube insertion. (From Roberts JR, Hedges JR: Clinical Procedures in Emergency Medicine, ed 4, Philadelphia, WB Saunders, 2004, with permission.)

5. Use your finger to confirm that you are through the pleural wall; usually you can feel the lung.
6. Clamp the chest tube with the Kelly clamp, and insert the tube into the pleural cavity using the clamp, generally aiming posteriorly and toward the apex of the chest as displayed in Figure 12-9.
7. Remove the Kelly clamp when the tube is in the thoracic cavity, and manually advance the tube further.
8. Clamp the tube with the Kelly clamp, and suture the tube in place to the surrounding skin.
9. Attach the tube to the suction unit.
10. Obtain a postprocedure chest x-ray to ensure proper placement.
11. When removing the tube, have the patient inspire maximally and hold his breath.

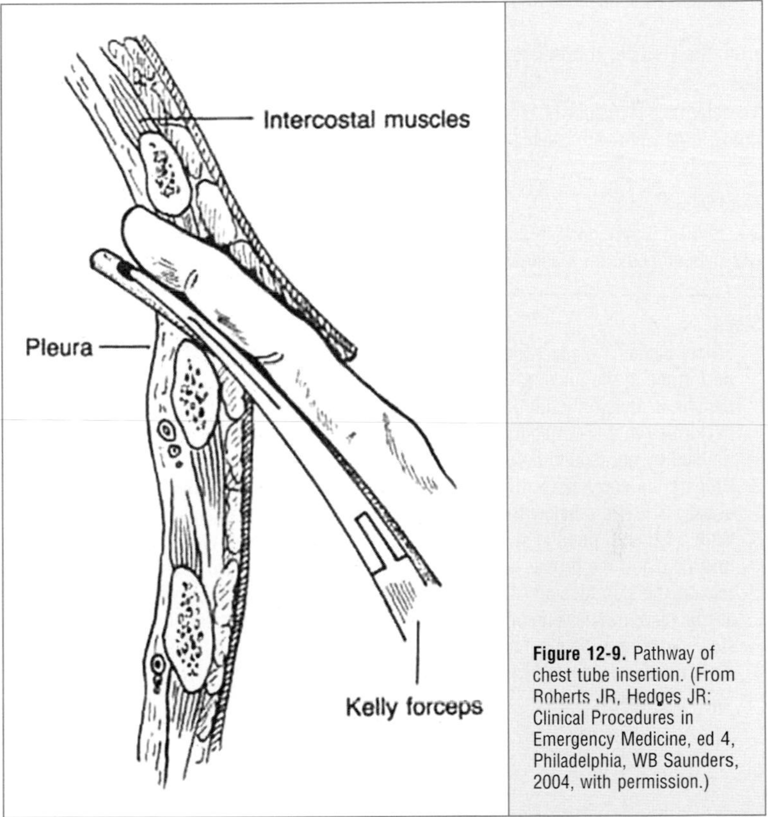

Figure 12-9. Pathway of chest tube insertion. (From Roberts JR, Hedges JR: Clinical Procedures in Emergency Medicine, ed 4, Philadelphia, WB Saunders, 2004, with permission.)

12. List the usage, necessary materials, and procedural steps of a thoracentesis.

Use

To determine the cause of a new pleural effusion (>1 cm on lateral decubitus view on x-ray) or to remove pleural fluid.

Materials

Thoracentesis kits often contain a 20- to 60-mL syringe and a 22-gauge needle, lidocaine.

Steps

1. Because the patient's back must be vertical, have the patient sit at the edge of the bed, with the head and arms supported on a bedside table.
2. Prepare the site with chlorhexidine and drape. Anesthetize with lidocaine.
3. Midway between the spine and posterior axillary line, use the chest x-ray and count ribs to where the effusion will be. Frequently, the site for thoracentesis will be marked by ultrasound before the procedure.
4. With the proper needle, enter the pleural cavity above the rib to avoid the neurovascular bundle that runs below the rib. Do not enter below the eighth intercostal space because of risk to the spleen and liver.
5. Aspirate the amount of fluid needed. For therapeutic taps, a catheter is often inserted over a larger needle.
6. As the needle is withdrawn, have the patient perform a Valsalva maneuver or hum to decrease the chances of a pneumothorax.

13. List the usage, materials, and procedural steps of a paracentesis.

Use

To determine the cause of ascites, to rule out spontaneous bacterial peritonitis, or for removal of fluids in patients with ascites for symptomatic relief.

Materials

20- to 60-mL syringe, 1.5-inch steel needle or blunt steel cannula with removable stylet (22-gauge needle for diagnostic taps, 16-gauge for therapeutic taps), lidocaine.

Steps

1. Empty patient's bladder. Patient with tense ascites may be placed supine with the tap performed in the midline. Patients with less ascites can be placed either in the lateral decubitus position (with the tap performed in the midline) or supine (with the tap performed in a lower abdominal quadrant). Frequently, the location for the puncture will be marked by ultrasound before the paracentesis.
2. Prepare the entry site with iodine solution and apply sterile drapes. The insertion site is usually 3 to 4 cm below the umbilicus. Anesthetize with lidocaine.
3. With one hand, pull the skin down 2 cm from insertion site. With the other hand, enter the midline using the proper needle at the insertion site. Once the needle has pierced the skin, release the skin tension (this is called the Z-technique, which creates a track to prevent ascitic fluid from leaking once the procedure is complete) and continue to advance the needle slowly in 5-mm increments, aspirating intermittently until fluid returns.
4. Aspirate fluid for tests or therapy as displayed in Figure 12-10, *B*.

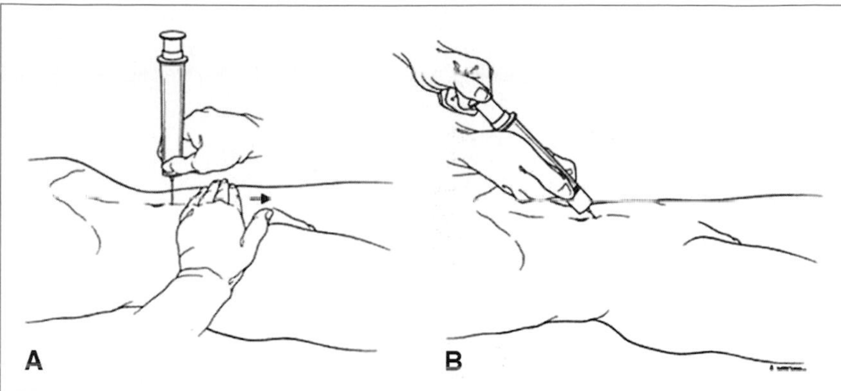

Figure 12-10. Aspiration of fluid during a paracentesis. (From Roberts JR, Hedges JR: Clinical Procedures in Emergency Medicine, ed 4, Philadelphia, WB Saunders, 2004, with permission.)

KEY POINTS: PROCEDURES

1. Medical students will be expected to be able to perform a variety of procedures. Be sure to follow all standard barrier precautions and note that most procedures require proper supervision.
2. Before a blood draw for an arterial blood gas measurement, verify artery patency of the collateral circulation with the Allen test.
3. Before removing a Foley catheter be sure to deflate the balloon.
4. When performing a procedure that involves invasive needles, it is common to anesthetize the skin using lidocaine.
5. When inserting the needle for a paracentesis, use the Z-technique to create a track that prevents postprocedure fluid leakage.

APPENDIX A

HISTORY TAKING

Derek K. Juang and Mitesh S. Patel

1. List the components of the Glasgow Coma Scale (GCS).

TABLE A-1. GLASGOW COMA SCALE

Eye Response (E)	Verbal Response (V)	Motor Response (M)
1 = No response	1 = No response	1 = No response to pain
2 = Open to pain	2 = Incomprehensible sounds	2 = Decerebrate (extend) to pain
3 = Open to verbal command	3 = Inappropriate responses	3 = Decorticate (flex) to pain
4 = Open spontaneously	4 = Disoriented, converses	4 = Withdrawal from pain
	5 = Oriented, converses	5 = Localizes to pain
		6 = Obeys verbal command

2. List the components of the Folstein Mini-Mental Status examination.

TABLE A-2. FOLSTEIN MINI-MENTAL STATUS EXAMINATION

Maximum Score	
5	What time is it (year, season, month, day, date)?
5	Where are we (state, country, town, hospital, floor)?
3	Examiner names 3 objects. Ask patient to repeat all 3. Give 1 point for each correct answer.
5	Serial 7's from 100 to 65 (1 point for each answer), or spell "world" backwards.
3	Ask again to recall 3 objects named above
2	Examiner points to 2 common objects (e.g., pencil, watch) and patient names them.
1	Repeat the following: "No ifs, ands, or buts."
3	Follow three-step command: "Take the paper in your right hand, fold it in half, and place it on the floor."
1	Read and obey the following: CLOSE YOUR EYES
1	Write a sentence.
1	Copy design.

3. What is included in a psychiatric mental status examination?

TABLE A-3. PSYCHIATRIC MENTAL STATUS EXAMINATION

Category	Description
Appearance	Try to give a complete verbal picture of the patient, including age, dress, posturing, grooming, eye contact, etc.
Speech	Volume, rate, tone.
Motor activity	Rate (e.g., agitated, slowed), purposefulness.
Mood	How is patient feeling, usually put in quotes (e.g., "sad")?
Affect	Outward manifestation of mood (e.g., full, neutral, constricted, blunted, flat), and also whether or not it is appropriate to the patient's stated mood.
Thought process	Organization of a person's thoughts (e.g., logical/linear, circumstantial, tangential, loose associates, flight of ideas, thought blocking).
Thought content	Does patient have any suicidality? Homicidality? Paranoia? Delusions? Ideas of reference? Obsessions? Compulsions? If there is suicidal or homicidal ideation, is there a plan or intent? Any hallucinations or illusions?
Cognitive	Level of alertness and orientation.
Insight	How well does patient recognize his own level of illness (e.g., poor, limited, fair, good?
Judgment	How is patient's ability to understand facts and draw conclusions?

4. What is included in a geriatric assessment of functional status?

Activities of Daily Living (ADLs)

These are the essential elements of self-care; inability to independently perform even one activity may indicate a need for supportive services. Ask the patient if assistance is required for: bathing, dressing, toileting, transfering, grooming, or feeding.

Instrumental Activities of Daily Living (IADLs)

These are associated with independent living in the community and provide a basis for considering the type of services necessary to maintain independence. Ask the patient if assistance is ever required for administering his or her own medications, grocery shopping, preparing meals, driving, using other transportation, using the telephone, or handling finances, housekeeping, or laundry.

Other Issues

Assess whether the patient is safe at home. Are there stairs? Has the patient ever fallen at home? Is he or she able to call for help or if there is an emergency?

5. What additional information should be included with pediatric patients?

Perinatal and Neonatal Information

This is more pertinent with infant patients: Review birth date, weight, type of delivery, Apgar scores, age of mother, length of gestation, and the occurrence of any complications during and after pregnancy including jaundice, respiratory distress, or feeding problems.

Nutrition
For infants, are they being breast or bottle fed? If formula is used, what type? Is child receiving any vitamin supplementation? For older patients, what is their regular diet like? Are there significant amounts of soda or juice?

Developmental History
Has the patient reached all developmental milestones? Look for evidence of proper gross motor, fine motor, social, and language skills development.

Habits and Personality
How much sleep does the patient usually get? Are there any issues with regard to behavior?

Immunization
Ensure that the patient's immunizations are up to date.

6. What additional information should be obtained during obstetrics/gynecologic visits?

Menstrual History
Last menses? Are periods regular? Heavy bleeding with menses? Any chance the patient could be pregnant? How many days between periods, and how long do they usually last?

Pregnancies
How many previous pregnancies? How many live-birth deliveries? Any abortions or miscarriages? What types of deliveries (vaginal or cesarean)? Have there been any complications, including diabetes or high blood pressure? Any heavy bleeding after delivery?

Contraception
Is patient using birth control? What methods?

Health Maintenance
When was the last Pap smear? When was the last mammogram? Any abnormalities found? Ever had a sexually transmitted disease? Ever had pelvic inflammatory disease?

Family History
In addition to other diseases, ask specifically about breast and ovarian cancer.

NEUROLOGIC EXAMINATION

Derek K. Juang and Mitesh S. Patel

1. How are the cranial nerves evaluated?

TABLE B-1. CRANIAL NERVE EXAMINATION

Cranial Nerve	Description of Testing Methods
I (Olfactory)	Not always tested, but ask patient to recognize familiar odors such as coffee.
II (Optic)	Test visual acuity, funduscopic examination of each eye.
III (Oculomotor)	Test extraocular eye movements, papillary constriction, and accommodation.
IV (Trochlear)	Test extraocular eye movements.
V (Trigeminal)	Test facial sensation, jaw opening, bite strength. If patient is comatose, test corneal reflex.
VI (Abducens)	Test extraocular eye movements.
VII (Facial)	Testing voluntary facial movements: frowning, smiling, wrinkling forehead, and puffing cheeks. May also test strength of eyelid closure.
VIII (Vestibulocochlear)	Test auditory acuity of each ear. Romberg test also evaluates cranial nerve VIII. If comatose, may evaluate oculocephalic reflex (doll's eye maneuver).
IX (Glossopharyngeal)	Test palate elevation and swallowing.
X (Vagus)	If comatose, test gag reflex.
XI (Accessory)	Test lateral head rotation, neck flexion, and shoulder shrug.
XII (Hypoglossal)	Test tongue protrusion and strength on lateral deviation.

2. How is sensation evaluated?

Sensation should be evaluated at different dermatomes.

1. Test pain/temperature, vibratory, and proprioceptive (Romberg test, joint position) sensation.
2. Compare to contralateral side.
3. Test two-point discrimination.

3. **Locate various dermatomes.**

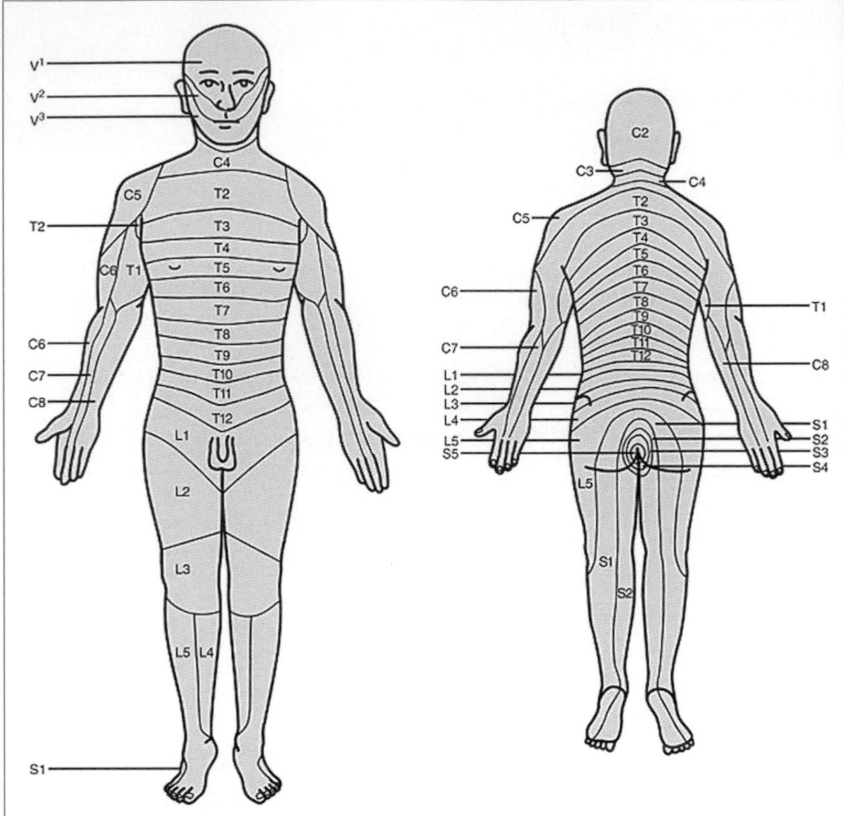

Figure B-1. Dermatome distribution. (From Wein AJ, Kavoussi LR, Novick AC, Partin AW: Campbell-Walsh Urology, ed 9. Philadelphia, WB Saunders, 2007, with permission.)

4. **How is strength evaluated and graded?**
   Test all extremity muscle groups and compare to contralateral side.
   Grading:
   5/5 Movement against gravity with full resistance
   4/5 Movement against gravity with some resistance
   3/5 Movement against gravity
   2/5 Movement with gravity eliminated
   1/5 Visible or palpable muscle contraction but no movement
   0 No muscle contraction

5. **Which reflexes are regularly evaluated?**
   Test biceps, brachioradialis, triceps, patellar, Achilles, and plantar reflexes. Compare with contralateral side.
   Grading:
   4+ Hyperactive with clonus
   3+ Hyperactive
   2+ Normal
   1+ Hypoactive
   0 No reflex

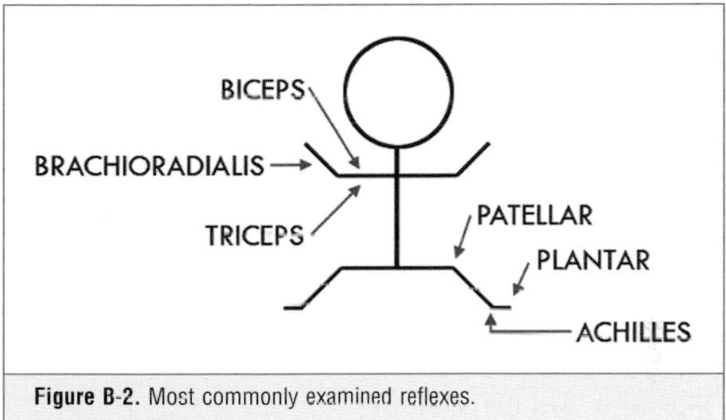

Figure B-2. Most commonly examined reflexes.

6. **List tests used to evaluate cerebellar function.**
   Finger-to-nose, heel-to-shin, and rapid alternating hand movements

7. **Which tests are used to evaluate gait?**
   Tandem gait (heel-to-toe), walking on toes, and walking on heels

APPENDIX C

MISCELLANEOUS

Derek K. Juang and Mitesh S. Patel

1. What equations are commonly used on the wards?

Anion Gap

$Na - (Cl + HCO_3)$
Normal = 10–14

FeNa

$FENa = [(U_{Na} \times S_{Cr})/(S_{Na} \times U_{cr})] \times 100$
U = urine
S = serum

Maintenance Fluids

Per hour, a person needs:
4 mL/kg for the first 10 kg (0–10 kg)
2 mL/kg for the next 10 kg (10–20 kg)
1 mL/kg for the remaining kg (>20 kg)

Creatinine Clearance

$[(140 - age) \times (weight\ in\ kg)]/(72 \times S_{Cr})$ for males. Multiply by 0.85 for females.
Note: This estimate is useful only if serum creatinine is not changing rapidly.

Alveolar-arterial Gradient

$[713 \times (FIO_2) - (PaCO_2/0.8)] - PaO_2$
Normal <20

Mean Arterial Pressure (MAP)

$(2/3) \times diastolic + (1/3) \times systolic$

Osmolality (estimated)

$(2 \times Na) + (glucose/18) + (BUN/2.8)$
Normal = 290 mOsm

2. **What is APGAR scoring?**
The APGAR scoring examination is used to describe the condition of newborn infants. It is determined at 1 and 5 minutes after birth. The score is the sum of five assessments, ranging from 0 (worst) to 10 (best).

TABLE C-1. APGAR SCORING

Appearance 2 = Entire body pink 1 = Pink body with blue extremities 0 = Entire body blue/pale	**A**ctivity 2 = Active movement 1 = Some movement 0 = Limp
Pulse 2 = >100 bpm 1 = <100 bpm 0 = Absent	**R**espirations 2 = Strong, crying 1 = Slow, irregular 0 = Absent
Grimace 2 = Cough or vigorous cry 1 = Grimace or slight cry 0 = No response	

3. **What composes the various intravenous fluids?**

TABLE C-2. INTRAVENOUS REPLACEMENT FLUIDS

Fluid	Na (mEq/L)	K (mEq/L)	Cl (mEq/L)	HCO_3 (mEq/L)	Ca (mEq/L)	Calories (kcal/L)	Glucose (g/L)
½ NS	77	—	77	—	—	—	—
NS	154	—	154	—	—	—	—
D5W	—	—	—	—	—	170	50
D10W	—	—	—	—	—	340	100
LR	130	4	109	28	3	9	—

D5W, 5% Dextrose in water; *D10W*, 10% dextrose in water; *LR*, lactated Ringer's solution; *NS*, normal saline.

4. **List the normal laboratory values.**

TABLE C-3. NORMAL LABORATORY VALUES

Blood, Plasma, Serum	Reference Range	SI Reference Intervals
ALT (alanine aminotransferase)	10–40 U/L	10–40 U/L
Amylase	27–131 U/L	27–131 U/L
AST (aspartate aminotransferase)	10–30 U/L	10–30 U/L
Bilirubin (total)	0.3–1.2 mg/dL	5–21 μmol/L
Bilirubin (direct)	0.0–0.2 mg/dL	0–3.4 μmol/L
Calcium	8.6–10.0 mg/dL	2.15–2.50 mmol/L
C-reactive protein	68–8200 ng/mL	68–8200 μg/L
Creatinine	0.7–1.3 mg/dL	62–115 μmol/L
Electrolytes		
Sodium	136–146 mEq/L	136–146 mEq/L
Chloride	98–106 mEq/L	98–106 mEq/L
Potassium	3.5–5.1 mEq/L	3.5–5.1 mEq/L
Bicarbonate	22–29 mEq/L	22–29 mEq/L
Gases, arterial blood (room air)		
Po_2	83–108 mmHg	11.0–14.4 kPa
Pco_2	35–48 mmHg	4.66–6.38 kPa
pH	7.35–7.45	[H+] 36–44 nmol/L
Glucose, serum	74–106 mg/dL	4.1–5.9 mmol/L
Growth hormone	0–4 ng/mL	0–4 ng/mL
Haptoglobin	26–85 mg/dL	260–1850 mg/L
Osmolality, serum	275–295 mOsm/kg	275–295 mOsm/kg
Phosphatase (alkaline)	25–100 U/L	25–100 U/L
Phosphorus	2.7–4.5 mg/dL	0.87–1.45 mmol/L
Proteins, serum		
Total	6.4–8.3 g/dL	64–83 g/L
Albumin	3.5–5.0 g/dL	35–50 g/L
Blood urea nitrogen (BUN)	6–20 mg/dL	2.1–7.1 mmol urea/L
Uric acid, serum	3.5–7.2 mg/dL	0.21–0.42 mmol/L
Cerebrospinal fluid (CSF)		
Glucose	40–70 mg/dL	2.2–3.9 mmol/L
Proteins, total	15–45 mg/dL	150–450 mg/L
Hematologic		
Erythrocyte count	M: 4.3–5.7 million/mm^3	4.3–5.7 × 10^{12}/L
	F: 3.8–5.1 million/mm^3	3.5–5.1 × 10^{12}/L
Hematocrit	M: 39–49%	0.39–0.49
	F: 35–45%	0.35–0.45

(Continued)

TABLE C-3. NORMAL LABORATORY VALUES (CONTINUED)

Blood, Plasma, Serum	Reference Range	SI Reference Intervals
Hemoglobin, blood	M: 13.5–17.5 g/dL	2.09–2.71 mmol/L
	F: 12.0–16.0 g/dL	1.86–2.48 mmol/L
Hemoglobin, plasma	<3 mg/dL	<0.47 μmol/L
Mean corpuscular hemoglobin	26–34 pg/cell	0.40–0.53 fmol/cell
Platelet count	150,000–450,000/mm^3	150–450 × 10^9/L
Prothrombin time	11–16 seconds	11–16 seconds
Reticulocyte count	0.5–1.5% of red cells	0.005–0.015
Sedimentation rate, erythrocyte	M: 0–15 mm/h	0–15 mm/h
	F: 0–20 mm/h	0–20 mm/h
Leukocyte count and differential		
Leukocyte count	4,500–11,000/mm^3	4.5–11.0 × 10^9/L
Segmented neutrophils	54–62%	0.54–0.62
Band forms	3–5%	0.03–0.05
Eosinophils	1–3%	0.01–0.03
Basophils	0–0.75%	0–0.0075
Lymphocytes	23–33%	0.23–0.33
Monocytes	3–7%	0.03–0.07
Drugs		
Acetaminophen	Therapeutic: 10–30 μg/mL	66–109 μmol/L
	Toxic: >200 μg/mL	>1,324 μmol/L
Vancomycin	Therapeutic: 5–10 μg/mL	3–7 μmol/L
	Toxic: >80–100 μg/mL	>55–69 μmol/L
Valproic acid	Therapeutic: 50–100 mg/mL	347–693 mmol/L
	Toxic: >100 μg/mL	>693 μmol/L

F, Female; *M*, male.
Values are for adults and may vary by institution. Unless specified, values are for male patients.
From Goldman L, Ausiello D: Cecil Medicine, ed 23. Philadelphia, WB Saunders, 2008.

COMMON ABBREVIATIONS USED IN MEDICINE

AAA	abdominal aortic aneurysm
ABG	arterial blood gas
ABI	ankle brachial index
ABX	antibiotics
ACLS	advanced cardiac life support
ACS	acute coronary syndrome
AD LIB	as desired
ADL	activities of daily living
AED	automatic external defibrillator; antiepileptic drug
AFB	acid fast bacterium
AFP	α-fetoprotein
AIN	acute interstitial nephritis
AKA	above knee amputation
ALL	acute lymphocytic leukemia
AMA	against medical advice
AML	acute myelogenous leukemia
ANC	absolute neutrophil count
AP	anteroposterior
ARB	angiotensin receptor blocker
ARDS	adult respiratory distress syndrome
ARF	acute renal failure
AS	aortic stenosis; ankylosing spondylitis
ASA	aspirin
ATN	acute tubular necrosis
AVF	arteriovenous fistula
AVM	arterial venous malformation
AVNRT	atrioventricular nodal reentrant tachycardia
AFVSS	afebrile, vital signs stable
B	bilateral
BCC	basal cell carcinoma
BID	twice a day
BIPAP	bilevel positive airway pressure
BIVAD	biventricular assist device
BKA	below knee amputation
BMI	body mass index
BRBPR	bright red blood per rectum
BX	biopsy
CABG	coronary artery bypass graft
CAD	coronary artery disease
CAP	community acquired pneumonia
CCE	clubbing, cyanosis, edema
CDI	clean dry intact

CEA	carcinoembryonic antigen
CHI	closed head injury
CHF	congestive heart failure
CLL	chronic lymphocytic leukemia
CML	chronic myelogenous leukemia
CPAP	continuous positive airway pressure
CPP	cerebral perfusion pressure
CPR	cardiopulmonary resuscitation
CPS	child protective services
CRI	chronic renal insufficiency
CSF	cerebrospinal fluid
CTA	clear to auscultation
CVA	cerebrovascular accident
CVP	central venous pressure
CX	culture
CXR	chest x-ray
DBP	diastolic blood pressure
DC	discharge; discontinue
D&C	dilation and curettage
DIC	disseminated intravascular coagulopathy
DJD	degenerative joint disease
DKA	diabetic ketoacidosis
DM	diabetes mellitus
DNI	do not intubate
DNR	do not resuscitate
DPL	diagnostic peritoneal lavage
DPOA	durable power of attorney
DRE	digital rectal examination
DTR	deep tendon reflex
DVT	deep venous thrombosis
DX	diagnosis
EBL	estimated blood loss
ECG	electrocardiogram (also known as EKG)
ECHO	echocardiography
ECMO	extracorporeal membrane oxygenation
ECT	electroconvulsive therapy
ED	erectile dysfunction
EEG	electroencephalogram
EF	ejection fraction (in reference to ventricular function)
EGD	esophagogastroduodenoscopy
EJ	external jugular
EKG	electrocardiogram (also known as ECG)
EMG	electromyelogram
EOMI	extraocular muscles intact
ERCP	endoscopic retrograde cholangiopancreatography
ESLD	end-stage liver disease
ESR	erythrocyte sedimentation rate
ESRD	end-stage renal disease
ESWL	extracorporeal shock wave lithotripsy
EX LAP	exploratory laparotomy
FEV1	forced expiratory volume in 1 second
FFP	fresh frozen plasma
FNA	fine-needle aspiration

FTT	failure to thrive
FUO	fever of unknown origin
FX	fracture
GBM	glioblastoma multiforme
GBS	Group B *Streptococcus*
GCS	Glasgow Coma Scale
GIB	gastrointestinal bleeding
GNR	Gram-negative rod
GOO	gastric outlet obstruction
G#P#	gravida = number of times pregnant; para = number of live births
GPC	Gram-positive coccus
GSW	gun shot wound
GTT	glucose tolerance test
G-Tube	gastric feeding tube
GVHD	graft versus host disease
HA	headache
HAART	highly active antiretroviral therapy
HCC	hepatocellular carcinoma
HCG	human chorionic gonadotropin
HD	hemodialysis
HEENT	head, ears, eyes, nose, throat
HELLP	hemolysis elevated liver enzymes low platelets
H&H	hemoglobin and hematocrit
HI	homicidal ideation
HIT	heparin-induced thrombocytopenia
HL	heparin lock
HPV	human papilloma virus
HRT	hormone replacement therapy
HS	at bedtime
HSM	hepatosplenomegaly
HTN	hypertension
HUS	hemolytic uremic syndrome
IABP	intraaortic balloon pump
IBD	inflammatory bowel disease
IBS	irritable bowel syndrome
ICD	implantable cardiac defibrillator
ICP	intracranial pressure
I&D	incision and drainage
IJ	internal jugular
ILD	interstitial lung disease
IM	intramuscular
I&O	ins and outs (referring to fluids)
IPF	idiopathic pulmonary fibrosis
IRB	institutional review board
IUD	intrauterine device
IUP	intrauterine pregnancy
IVF	intravenous fluids; in vitro fertilization
IVP	intravenous pyelogram
J-Tube	jejunal feeding tube
JVD	jugular venous distention
JVP	jugular venous pressure
KUB	kidneys ureters and bladder
KVO	keep vein open

LAD	left anterior descending (coronary artery); left axis deviation
LAP	laparoscopic, laparotomy
LBP	low back pain
LCX	left circumflex (coronary artery)
LFT	liver function test
LMA	laryngeal mask airway
LOA	lysis of adhesions
LOC	loss of consciousness
LP	lumbar puncture
LR	lactated Ringer's
LVAD	left ventricular assist device
LVEDP	left ventricular end-diastolic pressure
LVH	left ventricular hypertrophy
MI	myocardial infarction
MICU	medical intensive care unit
M&M	morbidity and mortality
MMP	multiple medical problems
MRCP	magnetic resonance cholangiopancreatography
MRSA	methicillin-resistant *Staphylococcus aureus*
MSSA	methicillin-sensitive *Staphylococcus aureus*
NAD	no apparent distress; no acute disease
NCAT	normocephalic atraumatic
NGT	nasogastric tube
NIF	negative inspiratory force
NKDA	no known drug allergies
NMS	neuroleptic malignant syndrome
NOS	not otherwise specified
NPO	nothing by mouth
NSR	normal sinus rhythm
NTD	nothing to do
OA	osteoarthritis
OCP	oral contraceptive pill
OD	right eye
OLT	orthotopic liver transplant
OOB	out of bed
O&P	ovum and parasites
ORIF	open reduction with internal fixation
OS	left eye
OSA	obstructive sleep apnea
OT	occupational therapy
OTC	over the counter
OU	both eyes
PACU	postanesthesia care unit
PCA	patient-controlled analgesia
PCI	percutaneous coronary intervention
PCP	primary care physician; *Pneumocystis* pneumonia
PCWP	pulmonary capillary wedge pressure
PE	physical examination; pulmonary embolism
PEG	percutaneous endoscopic gastrostomy
PERRL	pupils equal, round, reactive to light
PFTs	pulmonary function tests
PICC	peripherally inserted central catheter
PID	pelvic inflammatory disease

PIH	pregnancy-induced hypertension
PMI	point of maximum impulse
PMN	polymorphonuclear leukocytes
PNA	pneumonia
PND	paroxysmal nocturnal dyspnea
PO	by mouth
PPH	primary pulmonary hypertension
PPN	peripheral parenteral nutrition
PR	per rectum
PRBCs	packed red blood cells
PRN	Refers to treatments that patient can receive on an "as needed" basis
PTCA	percutaneous transluminal coronary angioplasty
PTX	pneumothorax
PVC	premature ventricular contraction
PVD	peripheral vascular disease; posterior vitreous detachment
PVR	postvoid residual
Q	every (refers to a time interval, e.g., if followed by "6," means "every 6 hours")
QHS	every night
QID	four times per day
RAD	right axis deviation; reactive airways disease
RCC	renal cell cancer
ROM	range of motion
RRR	regular rate and rhythm
RSV	respiratory syncytial virus
RT	respiratory therapy
RUG	retrograde urethrogram
RVR	rapid ventricular response
RX	treatment; prescription
2/2	secondary to
SAAG	serum ascites albumin gradient
SAH	subarachnoid hemorrhage
SBE	subacute bacterial endocarditis
SBO	small bowel obstruction
SBP	spontaneous bacterial peritonitis
SC	subcutaneous
SI	suicidal ideation
SIRS	systemic inflammatory response syndrome
SL	sublingual
SLE	systemic lupus erythematosus; slit lamp examination
SLR	straight leg raise
S/P	status post; supra pubic
SQ	subcutaneous
SSI	sliding scale insulin
SSRI	selective serotonin reuptake inhibitor
STAT	immediately
SVG	saphenous vein graft
SX	symptoms
TAH	total abdominal hysterectomy
TB	tuberculosis; total bilirubin
T&C	type and cross
TCA	tricyclic antidepressant
TEE	transesophageal echocardiogram
THA	total hip arthroplasty

THR	total hip replacement
TIA	transient ischemic attack
TID	three times per day
TIPS	transvenous intrahepatic porto-systemic shunt
TKA	total knee arthroplasty
TMN	tumor metastases nodes (universal tumor staging system)
TOA	tubo-ovarian abscess
TPN	total parenteral nutrition
TRUS	transrectal ultrasound
T&S	type and screen
TTE	transthoracic echocardiogram
TURP	transurethral prostatectomy
TX	transfusion; treatment
UA	urine analysis; uric acid; unstable angina
UC	ulcerative colitis
UO	urine output
URI	upper respiratory tract infection
US	ultrasound
VA	visual acuity
VATS	video-assisted thoracoscopic surgery
VBAC	vaginal birth after cesarean section
VBG	venous blood gas

INDEX

Page numbers followed by *t* indicate tables; *f,* figures. Page numbers in **boldface** type indicate complete chapters.

D

E